HEALTH SYSTEMS RESEARCH

Edited by K. Davis and W. van Eimeren

B. Horisberger R. Dinkel (Eds.)

The Perception and Management of Drug Safety Risks

With 29 Figures and 13 Tables

Springer-Verlag
Berlin Heidelberg New York
London Paris Tokyo

Dr. Bruno Horisberger
Interdisciplinary Research Centre
for Public Health
Rorschacher Straße 103c
CH-9007 St. Gallen

Dr. Rolf Dinkel
HealthEcon Ltd.
Steinentorstraße 19
CH-4051 Basel

ISBN-13:978-3-642-74274-3 e-ISBN-13:978-3-642-74272-9
DOI: 10.1007/978-3-642-74272-9

Softcover reprint of the hardcover 1st edition 1989

2119/3140/543210 – Printed on acid-free paper

Preface

In the past two decades public debate about the risks, benefits, and safety associated with drugs has intensified. Public disputes over risks are brought to court when individuals seek compensation for health problems attributed to a pharmaceutical product. The issue reaches legislatures and regulatory agencies when consumer advocates seek to influence the standards of drug usage. Front-page news tends to focus on accidents or other risk events with drugs.

Drug risk and drug safety have become an important political issue. Drug regulatory agencies have been instituted, and their responsibility has increased. The approval to market a drug is dependent on a set of sophisticated studies executed according to strict protocols and scientifically defined criteria. Drug surveillance activities have gained recognition, and reporting systems to identify drug safety problems have been strengthened. The understanding and management of drug safety is, nonetheless, beset by doubts, disagreements, and disputes. Conflict occurs over the significance of risk, the adequacy of evidence, the methodologies used to evaluate and measure risk, the standards that guide regulation, and the optimal means of communicating risk information to the public.

An international and interdisciplinary conference, convened by Ciba-Geigy in the spring of 1988, was designed to explore these areas of conflict from every angle and to initiate a collaborative effort to address existing shortcomings. The meeting at Wolfsberg, a historic estate overlooking Lake Constance, was a continuation of previous Wolfsberg Conferences dealing with issues of health care such as cost sharing, technology assessment, and socioeconomic evaluation of drug therapy.

The 1988 conference assembled academic experts in pharmacology, epidemiology, risk perception research, risk communication, and regulatory affairs, together with representatives of 30 leading pharmaceutical companies from 10 countries.

The Council for International Organizations of Medical Sciences (CIOMS) was represented as well as an industry association, the International Federation of Pharmaceutical Manufacturers Associations (IFPMA). Leaders of the consumer movement and representatives of the media participated actively in the debate.

This heterogeneous audience reflected the conference rationale: that the management of drug safety and risk is no longer a concern specific to the pharmaceutical industry, but has gained a social dimension.

Speakers and discussants emphasized common concerns and showed a strong interest in a collaborative approach to addressing them. Multidisciplinary collaboration was recognized as the sine qua non of successful management of drug risks.

In Part I of this book the drug safety issue is put in the larger perspective of the worldwide public debate on technological risks in an increasingly industrialized world. Many people have become sceptical and frightened of advanced technologies. Risk acceptance, however, constitutes an inherent part of human life and is a prerequisite for the development of human civilization and culture. To balance risks against benefits, to define acceptable risk, and to exclude what no longer falls within this category remain perpetual challenges.

Benefit/risk assessment often leads to controversy because it involves both factual analysis and value judgements. Within a given country, different groups have different stakes in defining the risks and benefits of drugs and evaluating the acceptability of the risks and benefits. At the international level, cultural and political values and expectations influence the way in which potential risks are perceived, evaluated, and controlled. Several authors analyze the factors which influence public perception of risks and benefits and propose means of anticipating, identifying, evaluating, and managing controversy about risks to health. A concluding paper presents a brief analysis of the significance of the major drug issues that have occurred in recent years and demonstrates the extent to which these issues are related to either efficacy, information, quality, cost-effectiveness, or safety. Of these five categories, safety concerns are predominant in the assessment, appraisal, and communication of the benefit/risk relationship of drugs.

Part II deals more specifically with benefit/risk analysis and appraisal in connection with drugs. Several authors delineate the current status, limitations, and pitfalls of pharmacoepidemiology resources and biostatistical data interpretation. The data bases available today are not sufficiently comprehensive to show all possible adverse reactions to drugs. Computer-based medical records linkage systems could help solve this problem. A case study about public controversy and government intervention related to adverse reaction reports on a nonsteroidal anti-inflammatory drug demonstrates the vital importance of adverse drug reaction reporting and other epidemiological resources in establishing regulatory and public consensus regarding the safety of a drug. Two papers present results of recent surveys of physician and public perception of hazardous activities and pharmaceuticals in Sweden and Japan. One finding is that, by providing information to the public about the adverse reactions possibly associated with a drug's use, the public's acceptance of drug risks may be increased. Another interesting finding is that physicians believe that their patients require relatively little information regarding medication, while patients indicate that they expect fairly comprehensive information.

Regulatory decisions are affected by both scientific and social considerations. Analysis and assessment of risk and benefit must be distinguished from the evaluation of the data. Whereas analysis and assessment are processes in which the scientific components prevail (e.g., animal and human data bearing on the safety of medicines), the evaluation of the data obviously goes beyond scientific evidence. Social and political factors (e.g., patient group interests, the media, economic pressures, ethical concerns) play a major role, the relative importance of which varies from country to country and over time. In regulatory decision making, scientific evidence and individual perceptions are closely intertwined. Information is assimilated and interpreted in different ways by professional groups and the general public.

Media coverage about risk analysis and appraisal influences policy decisions and stimulates public interests.

"Identify with the people who take the risks, then people will identifiy with you." This statement expresses the concern of several authors in Part III. This section deals with the consumer's perspective on pharmaceutical risk. The industry not only needs to develop a much better understanding of consumer perceptions but must also develop more effective ways of communicating with consumers. The industry's overall good track record in providing "hardware" – medicines and other therapeutic aids – has not been matched by its performance in providing "software" – information that the nonspecialist can understand. The challenge for the pharmaceutical industry is, therefore, to ensure that the patient is properly informed about the therapy and the risk associated with its use. A willingness and ability to communicate are key to improving society's acceptance of risk.

Part IV comprises, in a standardized format, a number of specific collaborative drug risk evaluation and management projects to the international pharmaceutical industry. The proposals cover the themes dealt with at the conference: pharmacoepidemiology, risk perception analysis, communications regarding the benefit/risk relationship, and risk appraisal on an international scale.

In Part V of this book the organizer of the conference expresses the conviction that people have great expectations for action and improvement. He concludes by summoning the pharmaceutical industry to transcend traditional boundaries and to reach out more imaginatively toward the industry's ultimate reason for being: the preservation and improvement of human life.

Part VI contains the curricula vitae of the authors, a very extensive bibliography, and index sections on subjects and data sources for those who want either to follow a topic that the book itself does not use as a structural principle or to seek specific information.

Contents

Part IV: Responding to the Issues

Part V: Outlook

Part VI: Annex

List of Participants

Dr. Richard B. Arnold

Executive Vice-President, International Federation of Pharmaceutical Manufacturers Associations, Geneva, Switzerland

Dr. Michel Auriche

Head of Drug Safety Department, Rhône-Poulenc Santé, Antony, France

Prof. Zbigniew Bankowski

Executive Secretary, Council for International Organizations of Medical Sciences (CIOMS), Geneva, Switzerland

Dr. Edward A. Bortnichak

Director, Pharmacoepidemiology, Pharmaceutical Division, Ciba-Geigy Corporation, Summit, NJ, USA

Dr. Arno Brandt

Director, Institute for Medical Informatics, Basle, Switzerland

Patricia Brown

European Editor, SCRIP World Pharmaceutical News, Richmond, Surrey, UK

Dr. Philip J. Brown

Publisher and Managing Director, SCRIP World Pharmaceutical News, Richmond, Surrey, UK

Prof. Rudolf Bruppacher

Head of Pharmacoepidemiology and Drug Safety, Ciba-Geigy Ltd., Basle, Switzerland

Dr. Dennis M. Burley

Director, Centre for Pharmaceutical Medicine, Woking, Surrey, UK

Lesley Bygrave-Malin

Chairman and Managing Director, Medical Viewpoint Ltd., London, UK

Dr. Davide Canti
Medical Director, Ciba-Geigy S.p.A., Origgio, Italy

Dr. Paolo Capone
Director of Clinical Research, A. Menarini S.A.S., Florence, Italy

Peter F. Carpenter
Chairman of the Strategic Planning Committee, Alza Corporation, Palo Alto, California, USA

Dr. Michael G. Carter
International Medical Director and Board Member, ICI Pharmaceuticals, Macclesfield, Cheshire, UK

Dr. Dianne Chen
Head of Drug Safety and Vice Director of Clinical Research, F. Hoffmann-La Roche & Co. AG, Basle, Switzerland

Gary C. Cheng
Policies and Issues, Pharmaceutical Division, Ciba-Geigy Ltd., Basle, Switzerland

Dr. Thomas Christie
Vice-President, Medical Affairs, Wyeth-Ayerst International Ltd., Philadelphia, PA, USA

Willy Dierickx
Vice-President, International Public Affairs, Janssen Pharmaceutica N.V., Beerse, Belgium

Dr. Rolf Dinkel
Member of the Management Committee, HealthEcon Ltd., Basle, Switzerland

Dr. Jean G. Domenet
Head of Medical Department, Ciba-Geigy Pharmaceuticals, Horsham, UK

Dr. John Dunne
Deputy Director General and Chief, Pharmaceuticals, World Health Organization, Geneva, Switzerland

Stig Arne W. Ekedahl
President and Managing Director, Pharmaceutical Division, Ciba-Geigy Läkemedel AB, Västra Frölunda, Sweden

Dr. Roy Ellis
Senior Vice-President of Medical and Public Affairs, Ciba-Geigy Corporation, Summit, NJ, USA

Dr. ROBIN W. ELSDON-DEW

Director, Medical Services, Glaxo Group Research Ltd., Greenford, Middlesex, UK

Dr. ARTHUR J. EMMETT

Head of Central Medical Affairs Department, Pharmaceutical Division, Ciba-Geigy Ltd., Basle, Switzerland

MICHAEL FOLEY

Head of Communication Strategy Department, Pharmaceutical Division, Ciba-Geigy Ltd., Basle, Switzerland

Prof. GEORGES M. FÜLGRAFF

Scientific Counselor and member of several committees in the European Community and FRG

Prof. SHIRO FUJINO

Professor, Faculty of Economics, Chuo University, Tokyo, Japan

Dr. JUSTUS GELZER

Head of Medical Department, Pharmaceutical Division, Ciba-Geigy Ltd., Basle, Switzerland

Dr. BRIAN A. GENNERY

Group Medical Director (Europe), Lilly Research Centre Ltd., Windlesham, Surrey, UK

Dr. U. GOETZ

Journalist, Basler Zeitung, Basle, Switzerland

Dr. G.S. GOLDSTEIN

Vice-President, Medical Affairs, Sterling Drug Inc., New York, NY, USA

Dr. GARTH K. GRAHAM

Vice-President, Product Safety, Smith, Kline and French Laboratories, Philadelphia, PA, USA

Dr. HARRY A. GUESS

Senior Director of Epidemiology, Merck, Sharp & Dohme Research Labs., West Point, PA, USA

Dr. HANSPETER HAUSER

Head of Region Management and PIC Pharmaceutical Division, Ciba-Geigy Ltd., Basle, Switzerland

Prof. Robert Hess

Head of Toxicology, Central Function Protection of Health and Environment, Ciba-Geigy Ltd., Basle, Switzerland

Dr. Siegfried Hiemstra

Head of International Drug Safety Department, Boehringer Mannheim GmbH, Mannheim, FRG

Michael D. Holland

President, Pharmaceutical Division, Ciba-Geigy (Japan) Ltd., Takarezuka, Japan

Dr. Bruno Horisberger

Director of the Interdisciplinary Research Centre for Public Health, St. Gallen, Switzerland

Dr. S. Hubbard

Editor, Ciba-Geigy Journal, Ciba-Geigy Ltd., Basle, Switzerland

Leon Jacobs

President and General Manager, Pharmaceutical Division, Ciba-Geigy Canada Ltd., Mississauga, Canada

Dr. Armin M. Kessler

General Director and President, Pharmaceutical Division, F. Hoffmann-La Roche & Co. AG, Basle, Switzerland

Dr. Harriet Kiltie

Medical Director, Lederle Laboratories Division, American Cyanamid Company, Pearl River, NY, USA

Dr. Tadashi Kitaguchi

Manager, Pharmaceutical Information and Regulatory Affairs, Takeda Chemical Industries Ltd., Osaka, Japan

Prof. Jan Koch-Weser

Director, Clinical Research, F. Hoffmann-La Roche & Co. AG, Basle, Switzerland

Dr. Alex Krauer

President, Chairman of the Board and Managing Director, Ciba-Geigy Ltd., Basle, Switzerland

Prof. Pierre Krupp

Head of Drug Monitoring Centre, Pharmaceutical Division, Sandoz Ltd., Basle, Switzerland

Henner Lappe

Head of Marketing Research, Pharmaceutical Division, Ciba-Geigy Ltd., Basle, Switzerland

Prof. Louis Lasagna

Dean, Sackler School of Graduate Biomedical Sciences; Academic Dean of the Medical School; Professor of Psychiatry (Clinical Pharmacology); Professor of Pharmacology; Director, Center for the Study of Drug Development; Tufts University, Boston, MA, USA

Dr. Heinz Letzel

President, Staticon Gesellschaft für medizinische Forschungsberatung mbH, Planegg, FRG

Guenter Lewandowski

Head of Pharma Policy Department, Pharmaceutical Division, Ciba-Geigy Ltd., Basle, Switzerland

Dr. William W. Lowrance

Senior Fellow and Director, Life Sciences and Public Policy Program, The Rockefeller University, New York, NY, USA

Charles Medawar

Director, Social Audit Ltd., London, UK

Dana L. Miller

Policies and Issues, Pharmaceutical Division, Ciba-Geigy Ltd., Basle, Switzerland

Yuichi Mizutani

General Manager, Frankfurt Office, Yamanouchi Pharmaceutical Co. Ltd., Frankfurt/M., FRG

Elizabeth Moench

Executive Director, Public Affairs, Pharmaceutical Division, Ciba-Geigy Corporation, Summit, NJ, USA

Prof. Ruediger Mohr

Head of Drug Safety Department, Hoechst AG, Frankfurt/M., FRG

Prof. Dorothy Nelkin

Visiting Professor, Department of Sociology, New York University, NY, USA

H. Ohno

Journalist, Jiji Press, Hamburg, FRG

Jean A. Orsinger

Head of Pharmaceutical Division, Ciba-Geigy Ltd., Basle, Switzerland

Dr. Gwendolen D. Parr

Head of Drug Monitoring Department, Ciba-Geigy Pharmaceuticals, Horsham, UK

Beverly Peterson

Journalist, Associated Press/Dow Jones Wire Service, Zürich, Switzerland

Dr. Martin Pfeiffer

Head of Drug Safety Department, Bayer AG, Leverkusen, FRG

Dr. Jerome A. Reinstein

Director, Technical Research, Richardson Vicks Europe, Procter and Gamble Research and Development Laboratories, Surrey, UK

Dr. Roger Sachs

Vice-President, Regulatory Affairs and Clinical Safety, Pfizer Pharmaceuticals, New York, NY, USA

Dr. D. Sallière

Head of Drug Monitoring Department, Ciba-Geigy S. A., Rueil-Malmaison, France

Dr. Nelson H. Schimmel

Consultant, Medical Operations, Schering Research, Kenilworth, NJ, USA

Dr. Alexander Schultz

Editor, Medical Tribune, Wiesbaden, FRG

Takashi Shoda

Deputy Manager, Corporate Planning, Sankyo Co. Ltd., Tokyo, Japan

Dr. C. Siporin

Vice-President, Drug Development Corporate Medical and Scientific Affairs, G.D. Searle & Co., Chicago, USA

Dr. Peter Sjoestrand

Executive Vice-President, AB Astra, Soedertalje, Sweden

Prof. Paul Slovic

President, Decision Research, Eugene, Oregon, USA;
Professor, Department of Psychology, University of Oregon, USA

Michael R. Sonnenreich

Counsel, Medicine in the Public Interest, USA;
Senior Attorney, Sonnenreich & Roccograndi P.C., Washington, D.C., USA

Prof. Walter O. Spitzer

Professor and Chairman, Department of Epidemiology and Biostatistics, Strathcona Professor of Preventive Medicine, Professor of Medicine, McGill University, Montreal, Canada

Dr. C. Spriet-Pourra

Head of Drug Surveillance and Monitoring, Upsa Labs, Rueil-Malmaison, France

Dr. David G. Taylor

Head of Policies and Issues Department, Pharmaceutical Division, Ciba-Geigy Ltd., Basle, Switzerland

Dr. William E. N. Taylor

Head of Drug Safety Department, Boehringer Ingelheim Zentrale GmbH, Ingelheim, FRG

Peter G. Tombros

Executive Vice-President, Pfizer Inc., and Member of the Board of Directors, Pfizer Laboratories Inc., New York, NY, USA

Koei Uchida

Head of Pharma Policy and Public Affairs Department, Pharmaceutical Division, Ciba-Geigy (Japan) Ltd., Takarezuka, Japan

Dr. Robertus van der Giessen

Head of Central Product Management, Indication Area III, Pharmaceutical Division, Ciba-Geigy Ltd., Basle, Switzerland

Dr. Klaus von Grebmer

Head of Public Affairs and Corporate Issues Department, Ciba-Geigy Ltd., Basle, Switzerland

Prof. Walter P. von Wartburg

Member of the Pharma Management Committee, Ciba-Geigy Ltd., Basle, Switzerland

Dr. Harald Voss

Head of Medical Department, Ciba-Geigy GmbH, Wehr/Baden, FRG

Dr. Erwin N. Whitman

Vice-President, Medical Affairs, Pharmaceutical Research and Development Division, Bristol-Myers Co., Wallingford, CT, USA

Hitoshi Yamamoto

Director on the Board, Assistant to the President for International Business Development, Eisai Co. Ltd., Tokyo, Japan

List of Companies and Institutions Represented

Pharmaceutical Companies

AB Astra	Soedertalje, Sweden
Alza Corp.	Palo Alto, CA, USA
American Cyanamid Co. (Lederle Laboratories)	Pearl River, NY, USA
Bayer AG	Leverkusen, FRG
Boehringer Ingelheim Zentrale GmbH	Ingelheim, FRG
Boehringer Mannheim GmbH	Mannheim, FRG
Bristol-Myers Co.	Wallingford, CT, USA
Ciba-Geigy	Basle, Switzerland Horsham, UK Mississauga, Canada Origgio, Italy Rueil-Malmaison, France Summit, NJ, USA Takarezuka, Japan Västra Frölunda, Sweden Wehr/Baden, FRG
Eisai Co. Ltd.	Tokyo, Japan
Eli Lilly & Co. (Lilly Research Centre Ltd.)	Windlesham, Surrey, UK
G. D. Searle & Co.	Chicago, USA
Glaxo Group Research Ltd.	Greenford, Middlesex, UK
Hoechst AG	Frankfurt/M., FRG
Hoffmann-La Roche & Co. AG	Basle, Switzerland
ICI Pharmaceuticals	Macclesfield, Cheshire, UK
Janssen Pharmaceutica N. V.	Beerse, Belgium

Menarini S. A. S.	Florence, Italy
Merck, Sharp & Dohme Research Labs.	West Point, PA, USA
Pfizer	New York, NY, USA
Rhône-Poulenc Santé	Antony, France
Richardson Vicks Europe	Surrey, UK
Sandoz Ltd.	Basle, Switzerland
Sankyo Co. Ltd.	Tokyo, Japan
Schering-Plough Corp.	Kenilworth, NJ, USA
Smith, Kline & French Laboratories	Philadelphia, PA, USA
Sterling Drug Inc.	New York, NY, USA
Takeda Chemical Industries Ltd.	Osaka, Japan
Wyeth-Ayerst International Ltd.	Philadelphia, PA, USA
Upsa Labs.	Rueil-Malmaison, France
Yamanouchi Pharmaceuticals Co. Ltd.	Frankfurt/M, FRG

International Organizations

International Federation of Pharmaceutical Manufacturers Associations	Geneva, Switzerland
World Health Organization	Geneva, Switzerland

Health, Research and Consumer Institutions

Centre for Pharmaceutical Medicine	Woking, Surrey, UK
Council for International Organizations of Medical Sciences	Geneva, Switzerland
Decision Research	Eugene, Oregon, USA
HealthEcon Ltd.	Basle, Switzerland
Institute for Medical Informatics	Basle, Switzerland
Interdisciplinary Research Centre for Public Health	St. Gallen, Switzerland
Medicine in the Public Interest	Washington, D.C., USA
Social Audit Ltd.	London, UK
Staticon	Planegg, FRG

Universities

Chuo University	Tokyo, Japan
McGill University	Montreal, Canada
New York University	New York, NY, USA
Rockefeller University	New York, NY, USA
Tufts University	Boston, MA, USA

Media and Public Relations

Associated Press/Dow Jones Wire Service	Zürich, Switzerland
Basler Zeitung	Basle, Switzerland
Ciba-Geigy Journal	Basle, Switzerland
Jiji Press	Hamburg, FRG
Medical Tribune	Wiesbaden, FRG
Medical Viewpoint Ltd.	London, UK
SCRIP World Pharmaceutical News	Richmond, Surrey, UK

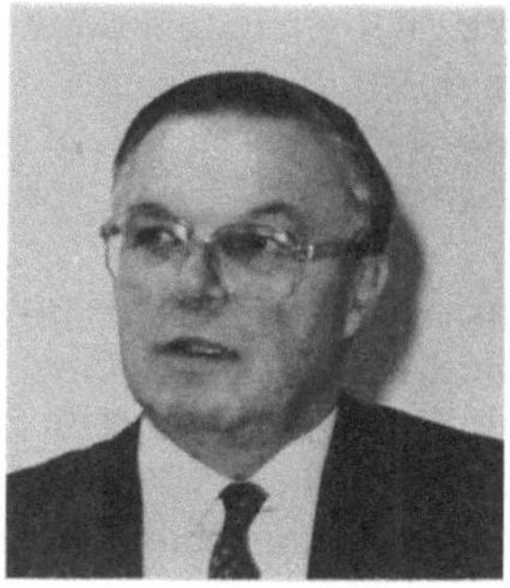

Opening Address

J. Orsinger

It is my pleasure and privilege to welcome you to our conference on "The Perception and Management of Drug Safety Risks". I would like to express my thanks and appreciation to all our guests for their interest and readiness to participate in this meeting, especially those who have travelled to Wolfsberg from overseas.

Our initiative in organizing this meeting has created an unexpected and overwhelming echo, and distinguished representatives and experts from scientific institutions, from about 30 pharmaceutical companies, from consumer organizations and from the media are present here today.[1] It shows that the issue to be discussed, namely "The Perception and Management of Drug Safety Risks", is a fundamental topic which not only concerns the pharmaceutical industry but is ultimately of concern to all those who in one way or another make use of pharmaceutical products.

Drug therapy and prevention bring daily benefit to millions of persons, but as we all know, every treatment with drugs is also accompanied by certain risks. All effective drugs bear some risks of unwanted effects.

Thus, the issue of drug safety affects us all. The debate over the benefits and risks of pharmaceutical preparations has reached a high level of intensity and is in part controversial. The need for consensus and common approaches to solving common problems has never been greater. There is probably not a single company represented here that has not at some time or another faced public questioning of the benefits versus the risks of one of its products. There is certainly none that can with confidence say that never, under any circumstances, will we be affected.

Public controversy about the safety of pharmaceutical preparations is not particularly new, but it has been gaining in intensity. Such controversy affects a company in many different ways. It is not merely a question of the product itself or of possible material losses. The impact goes much further, with a company's motives, image and reputation frequently being brought into question. There is also the damage caused to the confidence that is so essential between patient, the medical profession and the pharmaceutical industry. The new bottom line, in other words, is public acceptance.

If public trust and confidence in our activities has been dented, and there is some evidence that this is so, what can we do about it? Perhaps for a start we should follow the advice of the old adage, "physician heal thyself", and critically examine our own activities, constantly measuring them against state-of-the-art medical knowledge and

[1] See list of participants

opinion and against valid public expectations. The first step in regaining public confidence is surely to demonstrate competence in all that we do.

But simply amending behaviour is not enough; it is necessary but not sufficient. Actions may speak louder than words, but actions do not necessarily speak for themselves.

Hence we communicate, more and better than we have ever done before. This, in turn, necessitates an awareness of public perception, attitudes and opinions. Effective communication can only be possible when it is based on an understanding of public concerns and needs. Then, and only then, can a true dialogue take place.

Our conference will therefore try to examine and explore the key elements involved in therapeutic risk analysis, assessment, management and communication. Over the next few days, we will hear presentations from experts in these disciplines from around the world. We shall have the opportunity to listen to many different perspectives on the issue and to have a very open dialogue. Doubtless, we will not always agree, but the fact that we are here at all is a recognition of our concern, of a general desire to identify common ground and to take the initiative.

Ciba-Geigy has made a modest start in some of these areas and have embarked on an interdisciplinary program called RAD-AR (Risk Assessment of Drugs – Analysis and Response). I do not want to say too much about this here as the RAD-AR Programme will be introduced later this afternoon by my colleague Walter von Wartburg. Suffice it to say that RAD-AR represents the company's response to the challenges posed in this area of pharmaceutical practice. But it is evident, I think, that the issue extends much beyond Ciba-Geigy. If progress is to be sustained, cooperation in key areas will be essential. No one has a monopoly on wisdom; everyone has an interest in finding common solutions to common problems in the interest of the patient. At the end of the day, and I would like to underline this, it is the welfare of patients that counts.

The objective evaluation of benefits versus risks in drug treatment is an extremely difficult undertaking, and it is subject to considerable and varying judgmental interpretation. The present meeting will give us what I believe is a unique opportunity to address this complex issue in an open and interdisciplinary way, taking into consideration the opinions and findings of many experts. If our deliberations help us to make at least some progress in defining our responses and agreeing on ways of moving forward together, of finding some sort of common denominator, then I am sure that everyone will agree that the venture will have been worthwhile.

I wish you all an instructive, enjoyable and productive meeting.

Part I

Society and the Benefit/Risk Relationship

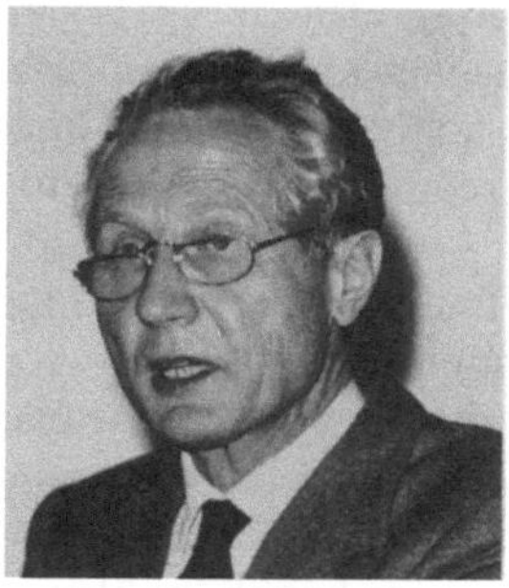

1. Acceptable Risk in Society

A. Krauer

Problems associated with drug risks and drug safety rank high on the list of priorities in discussions that are taking place within the profession throughout the world, and, what is more, the political content of these problems is growing. During the past 20 years or so, the public has become increasingly aware of these controversial topics. They affect the human race all over the world. Many people feel threatened, and many more are distinctly uneasy about them.

However, current discussions transcend questions of drug risks. They cover the full spectrum of risk/benefit evaluation in our world, where highly developed technologies tend to make an ever greater impact. Many people have become sceptical, and indeed frightened, of such advanced technologies as nuclear power, the manufacture of chemical products, biotechnological research and electronics; scepticism and fear are no longer confined to the young.

We know that we cannot simply turn the clock back on industrial development: mankind depends on science and even more so on technology and, in particular, on their continuing development, not only for the sake of survival but also in order to create and to ensure the long-term conditions for an acceptable quality of life.

Man's spirit of discovery and invention is such that it consciously takes risks – including unknown ones – in order to evade existing risks and to find new openings. Indeed, were it not for this readiness to take risks, human civilization and culture as we know it would not and could not have developed.

A human society which, on principle, opts for safety in the face of each and every risk would condemn itself to blocking all further development. In so doing, it would compel itself to remain at a standstill, and this, natural law teaches us, is tantamount to retrogression and final decay. Agreement will undoubtedly be achieved with relative ease on these basic positions. What will be much harder to achieve in each specific case is a clear definition of what constitutes the limits of acceptable risk, and what no longer falls within that category. Risk/benefit assessments will always lead to controversy because they do not only centre on rational or scientifically "provable" facts but also on questions of ethically justifiable responsibility. I believe we would be well on the way towards better mutual understanding if those holding different points of view in such controversies were to accept, or could be persuaded to accept, the fact that each position had been reached as the result of highly responsible effort on the part of an individual who had, in conscience, made the best possible use of all available knowledge.

Perhaps you will agree with me when I say: there is no basic disagreement regarding the direction that we should follow, but there do exist differing views as to the surest and most direct route that we should follow to reach our goal. I hope that our impending discussions will lead to a greater degree of agreement as well as to perceptible and tangible progress.

We are in need of this progress! I think I have made it clear that I am not advocating here "progress at any price". The ecological problems within our industrial society, so evident in recent decades, have shown us with utmost clarity that by no means everything which can be done should, in fact, be done. A degree of scepticism is appropriate here; keeping a certain self-critical distance is of the essence. But this must not go so far as to paralyse all our efforts to solve the immense health problems afflicting mankind. Far too great a section of humanity is starving without any prospect of being able to break out of this vicious circle. We are barred from taking the nostalgic road "back to nature". Thank God this is so, because we could not justify this, and it would ultimately have to be paid for by the poorest of the poor. This reason alone makes such a course of action totally unacceptable. This is why we must summon all available imagination and willpower as well as show much greater willingness for joint effort; otherwise, we shall be considered just as guilty as earlier generations that were not resolute enough in their fight against misery and injustice. Indeed, our guilt would be all the greater since we cannot seek absolution by pleading ignorance.

Industry, too, must face these major challenges. None of us must yield to the all too convenient temptation of adopting the course of least resistance or even toy with the idea of keeping industry out of potentially promising, but publicly controversial activities and functions in order to eschew the burden of having to justify making a corporate decision. That would be tantamount to cowardice, and we would be abdicating our responsibility for the creation of prosperity for the individual as well as for society as a whole.

However, industry can only make its best contribution if it is accepted by society and regarded as a credible partner. This, in turn, requires that it give proof of competence and professionalism, that it show transparency and ensure involvement and be open to all levels and groups of society, and, above all, that it display a credible willingness to undergo change. Only then will it be accepted; only then will it gain and maintain credibility and – on the basis of public confidence acquired in this way – make a successful contribution towards overcoming the challenging tasks of the future.

It will not be sufficient for us simply to draw attention to the indisputably great achievements made in the past by the chemical and pharmaceutical industries – achievements which have contributed so much towards the preservation and improvement of human life and the alleviation of human suffering. These achievements are well known and therefore, sadly, are now taken for granted. However, people do not judge us on the basis of our past merits – for this is "history" now – but we are assessed by our ability to solve present, and future, problems. To be sure, we must not shy away from self-criticism, but we must equally have full confidence in our ability to solve problems in daily competition with others. This means, above all, professionalism in our continual effort to live up to the most rigorous demands which the respective disciplines of our industry impose on us. This will enable us to reach in each case and at any given moment in time the highest standards achievable as well as cooperate in an innovative manner in their further development.

Based on such precepts, our discussions and decisions concerning the risk/benefit ratio of drugs, chemicals and other technical procedures and processes are not restricted to the domain of technical experts. Even the most highly informed expert will today find himself confronted with insoluble and insurmountable gaps in the data base, contradictory schools of thought and doctrines, and irreconcilable political positions, and he will have to operate and make decisions in a climate of virtual ignorance with little expectation of certainty. Controversial value judgements continue to haunt the artistic and scientific, medical and technical aspects of our industry. This inevitably exposes him to social and political scrutiny. Ever since the Renaissance and Age of Enlightenment, modern society has tended to make decisions and value judgements in a climate of uncertainty and to present these to the general public, instead of leaving this function to a select elite, to religious orders, wise men and so on.

Just as state authority, since the eighteenth and nineteenth centuries, has had to consider increasing demands for information and control, so areas traditionally left to the private sector, such as industry, will now have to consider demands for transparency and participation and accept pluralism of opinion and values. I am an advocate of pluralism of opinion and values. I am an advocate of pluralism for many reasons, but above all I support it because of its inherent innovative potential, and I believe that the decisive expression of one's own convictions in no way runs counter to this, but rather is its logical consequence. This maxim in no way seeks "government protection of vested interest"; on the contrary, it faces competition by means of competing concepts. This is precisely why it is more viable than historic "monopolies of truth".

Only in exceptional cases has progress been the result of dogmatic teaching. It will not, in future, grow out of a popularity contest with the spirit of the times, the so-called *Zeitgeist;* on the contrary, it will always be – and must always remain – the outcome of intensive work and effective striving for improvement. Nowadays, this process is increasingly taking place before the very eyes of the general public rather than behind the closed laboratory doors in universities or industry. However unfamiliar this change from backstage to centre-stage may be to us, and however challenging this may at first be felt to be, it must never be allowed to lead us to the erroneous conclusion that convincing proof of the correctness of our efforts can best be demonstrated by a withdrawal from this profession.

I am more inclined to see in this development an opportunity for new and genuine consensus. The closer we come to agreeing on what it is that we are ultimately engaged in, the more readily will research find acceptance (among the public). This, in my opinion, is the indispensable prerequisite for progress. Innovation, for its part, is a key element in ensuring the future and illustrates that engaging in economic activity is not an end in itself. This is as true of the economy as it is of health; those who live solely for the purpose of keeping in good health are by definition sick; health is a precondition for something else – it is not an end in itself.

We must cast aside all convenient models and so-called safe prescriptions of the past and devote our maximum efforts to the real task ahead: by virtue of our sympathy and empathy for human life, we must strive with the utmost diligence to preserve and improve its condition. People expect something to happen; they have great expectations. If we disappoint them, we will invoke their anger and resentment. In other words, our much vaunted professional competence would be seen as having let them down. Without convincing professional competence we will have no credibility, and without credibility there can be no trust.

If companies are, and wish to remain, an integral part of society, they must personify the principle of "responsible freedom". This means that industry must take very seriously those rules of the game which apply to all partners in every society and which serve to perpetuate the preservation of order in a free society.

In this context, great significance is given to the social and political framework within which economic and entrepreneurial activities take place. By using the metaphor "framework", I wish to refer, on the one hand, to those limits of the possible and feasible which the economy must accept and keep to; on the other hand, the economy must be given the opportunity of exploiting this "framework" in freedom and personal responsibility. The economy needs this creative freedom if its innovative potential is to be converted into concrete results. All of us, therefore, are dependent on the reliable and stable conditions within this "framework". Companies must bear their share of responsibility. Companies must bear their share of responsibility in the extent to which necessary controls are imposed on them by virtue of the way they are seen to use their freedom and carry out their responsibilities.

Anyone who knows our industry, also knows of its achievements and its efficiency and of those reserves that have hitherto remained inadequately tapped. We should feel impelled to mobilize these reserves. If we are successful in this, we will not only be able to achieve what society – to my mind rightly so – expects from us, but at the same time we will also be able to offer the world the most convincing justification for commercial success.

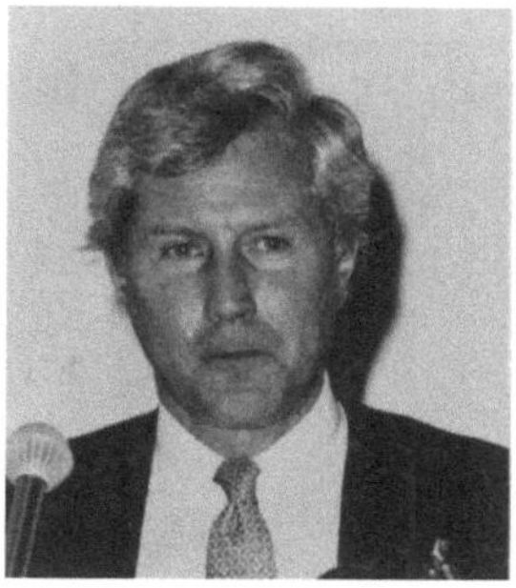

2. A Broad Framework for Confronting Health Risks

W. W. LOWRANCE

Throughout our lives we face a myriad risks to our health: fire, asbestos, barracudas, radon, earthquakes, nuclear reactors, automobiles, cholesterol, hepatitis ... Confronting all these threats is an ongoing personal agenda, both in the short term, as we plot how to cross the street or decide what to eat, and in the longer term, as we try to stave off bodily deterioration or catastrophe. Confronting them also is a core humanitarian concern and a central collective societal agenda, as we try to protect one another and seek fair distribution of risk burdens. The challenge always, of course, is to balance risks against benefits.

The purpose of this presentation is to propose a broad framework within which we can think about risks to health, whatever their nature. This will set the stage for evaluating pharmaceuticals.

The Concept of "Risk"

"Risk" is a compound estimate of the *likelihood* and *severity* of adverse health effect. Notice the two elements: likelihood (or probability) and severity (or magnitude). A particular risk description may be either relative or absolute. It may be expressed in a variety of ways. It may be derived from some statistical record, or it may be projected from testing or modelling. In all cases it must incorporate both the consequences and their likelihood.

To begin to bring order to the enormous and diverse array of risks that we face, we start by recognizing how they fall into categories. These might include the following (Table 2.1): infectious disease risks (such as influenza), life-style and occupational risks (cirrhosis of the liver), degenerative illness risks (cataracts), clinical risks (vaccine side effects), small-scale accident risks (sports injuries), large-scale technological risks (airliner crashes), local environmental risks (lightning), broad-scale environmental risks (urban air acidification), and catastrophic geophysical risks (tornadoes). Although they are informal and overlapping, these categories are familiar and can be very useful in sizing up and comparing risks.

Table 2.1. Types of risks

Infectious disease risks	Large-scale technological risks
Influenza	Dam breaks
Athlete's foot	Airliner crashes
Salmonella food poisoning	Toxic chemical releases
AIDS	Coal mine collapses
Life-style and occupational risks	Local environmental risks
Cirrhosis of the liver	Lightning
Cocaine addiction	Noise
Solar-induced skin cancer	Household radon
Textile workers' brown lung disease	Ragweed pollen
Degenerative illness risks	Broad-scale environmental risks
Cataracts	Stratospheric ozone depletion
Pyorrhea	Increase of antibiotic resistance in pathogenic bacteria
Alzheimer's disease	Urban air acidification
Osteoporosis	Agrochemical pollution of groundwater
Clinical risks	Catastrophic geophysical risks
X-rays	Tornadoes
Vaccines	Earthquakes
Hepatitis via transfusions	Volcanoes
Fetal damage in amniocentesis	Tsunamis
Small-scale accident risks	
Household fires	
Sport injuries	
School bus accidents	
Factory robot accidents	

My Core Theses

With a topic as ethically laden as this one, I think it important to state my assumptions:

1. Absolutely nothing can be absolutely risk free. There are no rewards in life without risk. Indeed, risk taking for benefit is the essence of human striving.
2. Decisions about risks involve both factual judgments and social (including personal) value judgments.
3. Risk-response actions should be viewed not as wasted costs but as investments that generate humanitarian returns. Approaching risk decisions as personal and societal investments is a powerful critical stance.

The Evolving Risk Agenda

It seems that as soon as we solve one problem, the newspapers announce another. This is emotionally frustrating, and it is frustrating to the conduct of public programs. For a number of reasons, risk issues evolve. Risk factors themselves – pathogens, intoxicants, technologies, exposures, vulnerabilities – keep changing. AIDS is a new pathogen; as far as we know, it simply did not exist earlier but emerged from biological evolution. As we alter technologies, the accompanying risks change. In the aggregate societal toll of illness and mortality, as any phalanx of risks is conquered others inevitably fill in. Reverend Malthus realized this in thinking about Dr. Jenner's new smallpox vaccine: as people were increasingly protected against the deadly pox, they would live to be vulnerable to other risks and would inevitably end up in other categories of the (also new) morbidity and mortality records (although later in life on average).

Scientific understanding of risks changes; obviously this raises new concerns. Practical possibilities of response – preventives, protectives, remedies, compensations – also change. And, further, the public's awareness changes, as do its values and priorities. People's worry-calculus evolves; risk-for-benefit judgments shift; so do ethical concerns, and the balance between being self-serving and sacrificing for others.

We must expect these changes, and we should prepare our institutions to accommodate them. For these reasons, too, the question so simplistically put by pollsters – "Is life becoming riskier?" – requires a lot of qualification before it can be answered.

Life-Enhancing Accomplishments

Profound achievements are evident if we look back over a moderately long period (between a decade and a century) in *Homo sapiens'* confrontation of risks. For most people everywhere, improvements in the basic conditions of life – food, water sanitation, personal hygiene, housing, energy, work environment, birthing practices – have substantially strengthened general health and resiliency. We have conquered a great many classical infectious diseases and other illnesses.

Further, we have learned how to deal with most acutely poisonous agents, solved most of the great malnutrition puzzles of the past, and learned how to defend ourselves against many accident and natural catastrophic hazards. Most acutely dangerous chemicals, metal-derived poisons (lead, arsenic), explosives, and mechanical and electrical hazards have been controlled, or at least made susceptible to control. Through precaution and education, countless everyday small-scale accident, sports, fire, and environmental hazards (lightning, sunburn) have been mitigated, or at least made more subject to personal choice. At the same time, medical screening and compensatory technologies have been devised against a formerly daunting variety of auditory, visual, dental, skeletal, hormonal, and other personal physiological deficiencies and stigmatizations.

The "bottom line", is that since the turn of the century, infant mortality has decreased markedly, and life expectancy has increased. On average, infants are getting a more robust start in life, and many more people are living longer, healthier, more vigorous lives.

Problematic Trends

Having improved our average lot so much, however, we are now encountering somewhat mixed blessings. In contrast to eons of crude survival-of-the-fittest, medical science is now preserving greater numbers of more vulnerable people. Increasingly, as we conquer the classic single-cause illnesses (such as polio), we are confronted by multiple-factor and life-style illnesses (such as cardiovascular deterioration); these causes are exceedingly hard to factor apart and analyze, and preventives and cures are hard to devise. Chronically debilitating, as opposed to acute, illnesses are becoming more prevalent, burdensome, and disturbing; this will be exacerbated as our society ages. Reproductive and genetic hazards are especially troubling because they affect people at the core of their personhood, are difficult to analyze and protect against, and may be perpetuated.

Furthermore, despite all those public-health accomplishments, the relevant sciences have entered what might be called a second adolescence. Pharmacoepidemiology is a good example; its basic statistical techniques have been developed to an impressively high degree and have been applied thoroughly to a few problems, but because of all the logistical, expense, and data-quality-control difficulties they are turning out to be hard to apply to the many other problems that demand their scrutiny. About many hazards, we now know enough to worry, but not enough to know exactly *how much* to worry.

Given all these trends, a dominant challenge for modern societies from now on will be the making of explicit, comparative, judicious choices among risk prospects.

Assessment, Appraisal, Response

Dealing with risks involves three separable modes of analysis and action. *Risk assessment* is the scientific or empirical description of the likelihood and severity of threat. *Risk appraisal* is the evaluation of the personal or societal burden from the risk, and of the costs required for protection or remedy. *Risk response* is the pragmatic prescription of "what to do about" the risk. These modes are distinguishable but interrelated.

The following elements must be built up to constitute the portfolio on any risk. They should be readdressed as progress occurs in factual understanding, social concern, or possibility of remedy.

Risk Assessment ("How much harm is incurred or is expected?")
- Characterize the hazard.
- Determine effects on individuals from exposure.
- Estimate individuals' exposure.
- Inventory the population(s) exposed.
- Relate degree of exposure to degree of effect (dose-response).
- Summarize prevalence, severity, and distribution of the risk in exposed populations and in society as a whole.

Risk appraisal ("How much should we be concerned?")
- Evaluate the personal and societal burdens from the risk.
- Estimate benefits and detriments associated with the source of hazard.
- Compare to similar risks and to risks from alternatives.
- Evaluate the costs and payback expected from protective investments.
- Consider ethical consequences of actions (or inaction).

Risk Response ("What should we do about it?")
Appraise practicalities in modifying the risks (technical feasibility and effectiveness, costs, political constraints, timing).
Decide whether and how to educate, warn, reduce, redistribute, or compensate for the risk.

Risk Appraisal

Little needs to be said here about the scientific issues of risk assessment; these are specialized for every kind of hazard; more will be noted below about the practicalities of risk response. But it is important at this stage to emphasize the pivotal power of the intermediating element, risk appraisal. Appraisal involves asking several critical questions.

In establishing importances or setting priorities, we ask: How prematurely – "before its time" – is the illness or death incurred? Does the risk affect children, for instance? Further, we ask: How preventable is the illness or death? If nothing can be done to prevent the harm, the issue may be moot. We try to take ethics into account. Are those who are suffering unfairly exposed? Are they unable to protect themselves? Is the lottery of life treating them especially badly? Can societal action of some kind help redress the unfairness?

We might perform a more elaborate risk-reduction investment appraisal, asking what cost must be paid per life extended or per risk altered. Or we might well examine several protective options, asking which is most cost-effective at achieving given protection. And in general we work toward gauging the benefit–risk balance.

Overall, we try to establish a context for acceptability judgments. Is the risk within the range of risks which society historically has been willing to bear? Is the risk borne voluntarily? And so on.

Comparative Evaluation

Countless sets can be defined within which to compare risks: causative mode (such as mutagenic radiation), societal function (electricity generation), geographic area (Basel), environmental medium (indoor household air), a population (anesthetists), product class (food colorants), specified illness, disability, or mortality (cirrhosis of the liver).

Thus, if we are concerned about botanical allergens, we might ask: Which pollens are the most aggravating? Concerned about electricity generation, we ask: How do coal mining, air pollution, and the other risks from coal-fired power plants compare against the uranium mining, radioactive waste disposal, and other risks from nuclear-fired plants? Or concerned about cirrhosis of the liver, we ask: What agents other than alcoholic beverages, possibly such as organic solvents, contribute to cirrhosis?

The proper formulation of comparisons, to which this paper will return, is of course crucial in the pharmaceutical enterprise.

Risk Response

For any risk a very wide spectrum of practical responses can be considered: investigate, inspect, monitor; restrict, contain, dilute; redesign; regulate, ban; inform, warn; certify or license practitioners; alter exposure, relocate; insure, indemnify; develop preventives, interventions, antidotes, remedies, or emergency responses; compensate financially for bearing. A correspondingly wide range of societal instruments can be drawn upon for effecting response. In many cases we depend on the market (such as for lawn mower safety features). In others we depend on standards of professional practice or on regulation (building codes), and in others on monitoring or insurance.

If harm actually is incurred, financial compensation for the damage can be provided through a variety of avenues, such as legal liability suits, direct compensation (such as coal miners' black lung benefits), or insurance. At present the pharmaceutical industry is reconsidering its relative emphasis on these various instruments of control and compensation. For example, it is reemphasizing consumer education and warning, is urging reform of legal liability structures, and is seeking robust indemnification against the risk gambles involved in providing new vaccines.

Perceptions and Attitudes

Papers by Slovic and others in this volume discuss perceptual research in detail. Here I propose a few of my own generalizations about people's attitudes.

Fundamentally, we in developed nations conceive of ourselves as risk-buffering societies. We try to protect each other, and we try to help those who are harmed. This is manifested in countless regulations that we have imposed on ourselves, in legal doctrines such as the duty of anyone who is aware of danger to warn those endangered, and in moral obligations such as parents' duty to teach children about hazards.

We strongly prefer to choose our own risks and resent having risks involuntarily imposed on us. We are more willing to allow others to undertake risky actions if the potential health and cost consequences are confined to the risk takers. Similarly, we are more willing to tolerate a risk in society if direct benefit accrues to those who bear the risk, or if those who bear the risk agree to accept monetary or other compensation from those who benefit.

Emotionally we find it easier to endure risks that fall on victims whom we do not know ("statistical risks") than on those whom we do know. And human nature tends to worry more about threats that are immediate and close to home than about those that are further away in space or time. Catastrophic, lumped losses (such as in the crash of an airliner) are emotionally harder to endure than a series of smaller losses (such as in automobile accidents), even if the smaller losses are equivalent in sum. Because as individuals our expertise and power are quite limited, we are as concerned that risk issues be supervised by competent, frank, honest, responsive, trustworthy authorities, as we are about particular risk outcomes. This has profound relevance for the pharmaceutical enterprise.

Ethics

Many ethical themes pervade risk issues, perhaps most noticeably questions of distribution of risk burdens and questions of decisional power. Here I would call attention to six themes that have to do with tensions between communalism and individualism.

Communal Commitment To Buffer Individuals' Risks. Fire protection is a venerable example; everyone respects all sorts of fire-prevention measures and contributes financially, via taxes or fees, to maintaining fire-protection capabilities; everyone benefits. As some government regulations and taxes exemplify, such collective efforts may be more enthusiastically accepted in theory than in implementation.

Joint Individual Risk Bearing for Communal Protection. Vaccination is a clear example; everyone in a group submits to the vaccine gamble so as to vanquish the pathogenic threat. (Schemes such as insurance and legal liability help compensate the vaccinated who suffer side effects.) As with the first theme, the communal and individualist objectives must be sensitively linked.

Protection of the Especially Vulnerable. Obvious examples include protection of infants, the elderly, certain groups of workers, and a variety of others who cannot fully protect themselves. Clearly these test our altruism – although, be it noted, everyone is especially vulnerable in at least several moments in his life.

Paternalism and Consent. As we try to protect those who are unlikely to or cannot protect themselves, issues of consent arise. Often paternalism conflicts with consent, such as in state regulations that people wear seat belts in automobiles, helmets on motorcycles, or hard hats on construction sites.

Communal Encroachments on Individuals' Freedom or Privacy. Regulation of traffic and highway speed, and mandatory screening for illnesses or narcotics abuse exemplify this problem. Public-health enhancements must be weighed against personal-space encroachments.

Self-Responsibility. Especially with respect to life-style habits that affect health, this issue is greatly increasing in importance. Society is diminishing its tolerance of self-harming behaviors and its willingness to compensate for self-preventable harms.

Sermon

Before moving to specifics in the pharmaceutical arena, let me summarize my thematic concerns. The following precepts should be applied in confronting any risk to health:

1. Distinguish between scientific risk assessment, social risk appraisal, and pragmatic risk response. Use appraisal to bridge between assessment and response.

2. Construe all risk responses as societal or personal investments. Invest only in those responses that promise substantial payback.
3. Characterize risks quantitatively, even if imprecisely. Estimate exposure realistically. Take special account of especially vulnerable individuals.
4. Express risks in decision-relevant ways, such as by normalizing for exposure. For perspective, develop relevant comparisons grounded in everyday experience.
5. Expect, and prepare to cope with, evolution of hazards, vulnerabilities, factual understanding, social valuations, and possibilities for response.
6. Use broad "scoping" appraisals to set strategic priorities. Use more detailed appraisals to evaluate the social payback from various risk-reduction options.
7. In reducing any risk, avoid merely transmuting it into other risks.
8. Whenever evaluating risks, evaluate related benefits, costs, and other attributes at the same time.
9. Over the long run, build up assessments of constellations of technologies or situations. Foster comparisons among major risk regimens.
10. Throughout, take ethical dimensions into account.

Pharmaceutical Risks

The Pharmaceutical Context. Let us take stock of the context. Drugs are deliberately targeted against specific health risks. They are, for the most part, voluntarily taken, and they are deeply experienced personally by consumers. The intended benefits of drugs are fairly clear, and they are susceptible of at least semiquantitative analysis. The acceptable benefit – risk expectation varies specifically by application and by user.

Unlike in many other enterprises, evaluation in this domain does not weigh risk against some broad benefit, but rather risk against risk. *The benefit of a pharmaceutical is reduction of risk impending from some health threat (influenza, hearing loss, whatever).* For any pharmaceutical, the crucial question is: Does the reduction in impending health risk achieved by the drug reasonably exceed any side effect risks imposed? The goal is net health risk reduction. In any such evaluation, inefficacies (the drug's failure to "work" adequately in some recipients) should be adjusted for. Inequities of outcome should be taken account of and addressed.

Failure of a potentially efficacious and low-risk drug to become available – pragmatically available to ultimate users – through lack of research and development, poor marketing, inefficient or improper use, over-restrictive regulation, or any other reason, obviously deprives potential net-risk reducers of the option. Unless other, equally beneficial protections or remedies exist, those potential users are left vulnerable to the impending health risk itself. Sometimes this point is overlooked as we strive so assiduously to minimize side effect risks.

A market complication for pharmaceuticals is that proxy consumers – doctors and other health care providers – make many evaluative decisions in behalf of the ultimate consumers. Another complication is that pharmaceutical issues increasingly are intersecting with those of over-the-counter medications, medical devices and diagnostics, medical biotechnologies, protective and restorative cosmetics, and nutritional supplements; managing these intersections will form part of the regulatory agenda in

	Therapeutic efficacy	Risk to patient	Costs (various)	Cost-effectiveness	Benefits (various)	Patient preference and ethics	Societal ethics
The drug of concern							
No treatment							
Alternative drugs							
Non–drug alternative							

Fig. 2.1. The pharmaceutical comparative matrix

coming years. Lastly, as is widely recognized, health self-determination by individual consumers is increasing in importance, as is health self-determination by nations.

Pharmaceutical Comparative Matrices. Ideally, for any drug we would like to have information to fill in the matrix of Fig. 2.1. Rarely do we possess all this information, at least with full reliability. However, such information is being increasingly developed now. As it becomes available, it is inducing major changes in decision making by doctors, patients, and health care institutions. As one thinks through the implications of this master matrix, which incorporates elements that implicitly, if not always explicitly, pervade medical practice, notice how the matrix reflects the central tenets of my "sermon": Compare; think appraisively; consider ethics.

Even wider perspective can be gained as depicted in Fig. 2.2. Drugs are a risk-reduction subset within the larger set of medicine (which includes health screening, dental and visual prophylaxis, and a wide range of other activities). Medicine itself is a subset within the much larger health care domain (which includes life-style regimens, health statistics, and other activities that are powerfully determinative but broader than classical medical care). And health care is a subset within the overall domain of health risk confrontation (which includes fire protection, disaster preparedness, and other activities beyond health "care").

For any drug, whether one already in use or one still being developed, the questions are: Is it the best drug for the application compared to other drugs? To nondrug medicine (such as surgery)? In a larger framework, does the application, say therapy, promise higher payoff to consumers or society compared to other health care investments (such as prophylaxis)? Then, in the grand framework, compared to other protective regimens (such as workplace safeguards)?

The first two of these questions tend to be raised in medical domains, the latter two in longer-term policy and economic domains. All guide the evolution of pharmaceutical development and application.

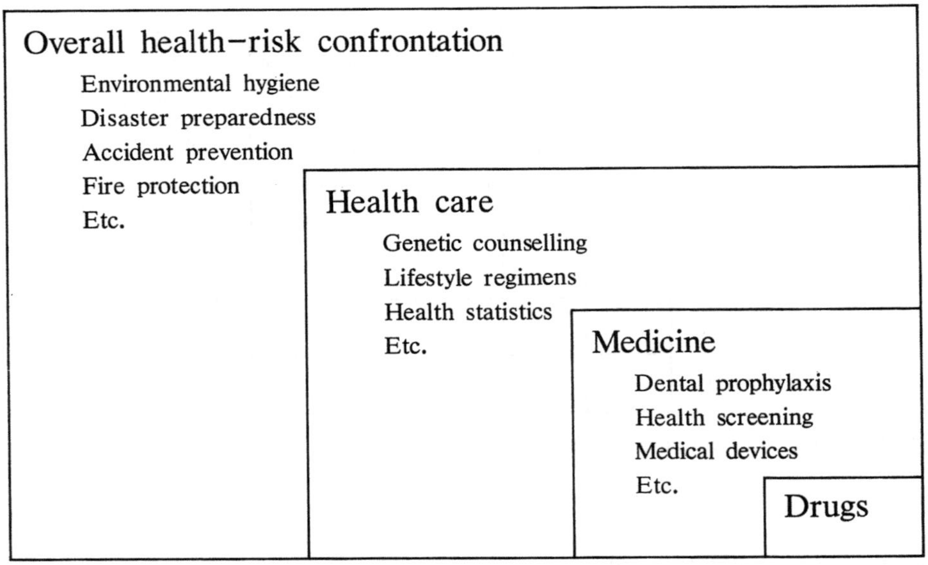

Fig. 2.2. Evaluative subsets

Confronting Health Risks

Much of the history of health and medicine has been determined by chance discoveries, cultural momentum, or the efforts of medical crusaders. Mostly, risks have been coped with on a risk-by-risk basis, with priorities emerging only de facto.

We must deal with health risks much more systematically and comparatively. Armed with critical new knowledge, anxious about budget stringencies, but ambitious to provide broad health protection to everyone, we now are squarely in position to confront the risks and to decide: to decide how to deploy screening tests; to decide which genetic risks to condone; to decide deliberately how best to spend public protective resources; to decide, where choices exist, between prevention and remediation; to decide between individuals' and society's obligations.

As we shift toward confronting risks strategically and attending more fully to ethical complexities, a robust framework of the kind proposed here will be essential.

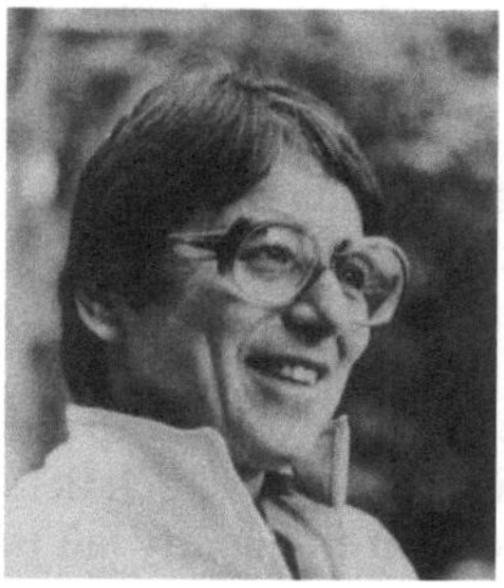

3. Communicating the Risks and Benefits of Technology: The Case of Pharmaceuticals

D. NELKIN

In the past two decades public concerns about the risks of technologies, ranging from nuclear power to pharmaceutical products, have been expressed in extended media coverage, frequent controversies, and increased litigation and regulation [38]. Risk assessment has become a veritable industry, involving the complex and controversial process of evaluating the risks of technology, communicating information about risks to the public, and developing appropriate controls. Evaluating risk requires interpretive judgment in the face of technical uncertainty and scientific disagreement. What constitutes significant and meaningful evidence? Whose judgment is to be considered in evaluating the severity and acceptability of risk? What rules of evidence should guide legal and policy decisions? Controlling and communcating risk involves questions of social responsibility and political legitimacy. What are the appropriate roles and limits of government in regulating industrial practices? What information should be conveyed to the public? Who should be involved in decisions about risk? These are deeply divisive questions and the source of heated debate, for risk assessments affect the economic interests and political values of different social or cultural groups.

Within a given country many groups have stakes in defining the risks and benefits of drug products and in evaluating their acceptability. The stakes are obviously high for manufacturers, concerned about the regulation of and market for their products, and for consumers, concerned about the effect of specific products on their health. But the evaluation of risk engages a variety of other "publics:" scientists, health professionals (including physicians, nurses, and pharmacists), health activists, lawyers, agency administrators, and journalists. Such groups operate from different frames of reference. Their economic stakes, professional ideologies, bureaucratic routines, career pressures, and political beliefs may all influence how they balance risks and benefits.

In different national contexts cultural and political values and expectations also influence the way in which potential risks are perceived, evaluated, and controlled. Thus, various nations differ considerably in the way in which they evaluate the risks and benefits of technology, convey information about risk to the public, and develop regulatory schemes [3].

The purpose of this background paper is to develop a set of guidelines for an international research project on the question of how various publics perceive the risks and benefits of pharmaceutical products. Risk communication is a critical aspect of this question. The paper analyzes risk communication as a social process on the assumption that there is far more to the communication of risk than simply the disclosure of technical information, and more to the response to risk information than simply technical understanding.

The first section will set out the context of the growing preoccupation with the risks and benefits of technology by indicating some characteristics of risk that must be considered in a project addressing the diversity of public perceptions in different social or national contexts.

The second section will review some characteristic research approaches to the analysis of risk and risk perception. In the United States this growing research field has been dominated by technical and managerial perspectives that frequently fail to account for the diversity of public reactions. Thus I will emphasize the importance of an approach that extends beyond the technical model to focus on risk as a social concept. In particular, I will argue that definitions of risk are an expression of the tensions inherent in given social and cultural contexts, and that these tensions frequently come to focus on the issue of risk communication.

The third section, therefore, addresses the social dynamics of risk communication in terms of two questions: (a) How do people know about the risks and benefits of particular technologies and products? (b) What is the influence of communication on perceptions, behavior, and public policy?

The final section will then propose a research agenda that follows from the background paper.

The Context: Attribution of Risk

Perhaps the most striking characteristic of "risk" in the 1980s is the extent of public concern that has been expressed in litigation and regulation, and in extensive and often dramatic media coverage. Public disputes over risk are brought to court when individuals seek compensation for health problems attributed to a technology or a pharmaceutical product. They reach legislatures and regulatory agencies when environmental or consumer advocates seek to influence the standards regulating the use of technology and to assure their implementation. They reach the press when accidents or other risk events turn technology choices into front-page news.

The preoccupation with risk sometimes reflects particular dramatic events: the Tylenol scare, the thalidomide crisis, the concern over the side effects of DES (diethylstilbestrol). Often such events become the focus of extended media coverage that tends to focus on tragic and frightening problems. But public concerns about technology extend beyond critical events to suggest a growing mistrust of both industry and government and of their ability to develop acceptable standards to assure the safety of consumer products. Mistrust is manifested in the popularity of dietary fads, holistic medicine, and self-diagnostic techniques. It is reflected in consumer behavior with respect to particular products and in the opposition to certain public policies (e.g., the swine flu vaccination program).

Apparent change in public perceptions of technology have generated a cottage industry of risk assessment, but it is an industry beset by disagreements and disputes. These reflect certain characteristics of technical risks that compound the difficulties of evaluation and leave considerable leeway for subjective factors to enter public perceptions. The nature and extent of risk are subject to technical uncertainties and scientific dispute. Uncertainties prevail at several levels: the extent and significance of problems, their causes, their potential health effects, and the appropriate methods of remedial action are all subject to diverse interpretations. In many cases, uncertainties exist because scientific information simply is not available. An exhaustive study by the National Academy of Sciences in March 1984 found that adequate information on potential health hazards exists for only 18% of 1815 pharmaceutical products, 10% of 3350 pesticide ingredients, 5% of 8627 food additives, and 2% of 3410 cosmetic ingredients.

Neither epidemiological nor laboratory studies can identify all the substances that may cause cancer, neurological problems, or genetic defects. Because of the limits of human experimentation, most laboratory studies testing the effects of chemicals or drugs must employ animals as research subjects, and their relevance to human reactions is frequently in dispute.

Even for intensively studied substances, the extent of risk may remain unclear, especially when health effects do not become evident for many years, or when risks are unlikely and therefore difficult to calculate, but could be catastrophic. Scientific judgments about risk are often constrained by inadequate evidence, relatively primitive diagnostic techniques, and limited understanding of the mechanisms by which hazards may affect human health. The cumulative and synergistic effects of multiple exposures to combinations of substances are poorly documented. Moreover, drugs and chemicals may affect different people in different ways.

It is hardly surprising, then, that specialists assessing risk arrive at divergent conclusions about the relative danger of particular substances and the need for regulatory controls [comprehensive bibliography on risk analysis: 6]. Conflict occurs over the significance of risk, the adequacy of evidence, the methodologies for evaluating and measuring risk, the severity of health effects, and the appropriate standards to guide regulation. Inevitably, conflict complicates the communication of risk information to the public.

In this context of uncertain, social, political, and economic factors enter risk evaluations. Although the concept of risk is often defined in the narrow technical framework of health and safety, it is more realistically viewed in far broader terms. Risk perceptions are embodied in complex systems of beliefs, values, and ideals that constitute a culture [10]. People predisposed to different values or forms of social organization will perceive different dangers. Defining risk can become a way of explaining the failure of existing political or social relationships, of voicing mistrust, and of delegating blame. These complex attributes of risk are reflected in the diversity of approaches that characterize the expanding risk assessment field.

Approaches to Risk Assessment

According to one estimate, the assessment and management of risk in the United States cost from 10% to 15% of the gross national product [4]. It has involved university researchers, consulting firms, specialists within industrial firms, and academics in disciplines including engineering, economics, law, and the social sciences. Their approaches, accordingly, have varied.

Technical Approaches

The field of risk assessment was first founded on several implicit assumptions: that evaluating risk is a technical matter to be resolved by developing better, more accurate scientific information; that there is an optimal way to characterize risk that reflects an underlying consensus among experts; that people fear technology because they are poorly informed or fail to understand the nature of risk; that they are misled by exaggerated media reports or hold basically irrational, antiscience views [see analysis in 19]. Thus public fear of risk has been frequently dismissed as "technophobia," and the American public has been criticized as "risk aversive," as "healthy hypochondriac," and as misguided or uninformed. If public fear of risk is defined in terms of inadequate information, then, it is assumed, increased technical evidence and better communication of this evidence by knowledgeable experts will allay public concern. Based on these assumptions, risk analysts seek a "rational" means to make decisions about technologies by developing quantitative measures through which to compare the risks of different choices, to calculate their costs and benefits, and to communicate these calculations to the public as the means to assure public acceptance of technological choices.

This technical approach guides government agencies, which evaluate risks by a process of hazard identification (e. g., monitoring the incidence of Reye's syndrome), hazard characterization (e. g., using case-controlled studies to confirm the association between Reye's syndrome and salicylates), exposure characterization (by surveying of exposure data), and risk determination (through evaluation of the data from various studies in order to reach a scientific consensus) [59].

Technical assumptions also guide the engineering and economic models of risk, including forecasting and systems-analysis techniques [21, 47]. Based on measures of mortality and morbidity, they seek to calculate in an objective manner the probabilities of a hazardous event, to identify the consequences for human health, and to estimate the likelihood of these consequences. What, for example, is a safe level of exposure to a chemical? What are the odds of an accident? What are alternative choices?

This technical approach to risk analysis is linked to a genre of policy research on the regulation and management of risk. These studies center on the policies and institutions through which controls are implemented. They include studies of the formal and informal decision-making process, the legal and legislative institutions of control, the setting of standards, and the ways of implementing regulations. Some examine the effect of interventionist policies, such as the banning of certain products, the restrictions on advertising, and the provision of public information in ways that will shape public perception [22, 31]. Others focus on the cost of controlling risk – "the risk of risk decisions" – in terms of money spent on reducing hazards and productivity delays [7, 52]. A related literature explores models of decision making that would reduce conflict in the area of risk and optimize the possibilities of legitimate decisions under conditions of uncertainty [see essays in 49, 58]. Their intention is to discover the relative effectiveness of various decision and communication strategies in order to "manage" the problem of risk. Their underlying premise, once again, is that risk is fundamentally a technical issue that can be accurately assessed and communicated to serve as a guide for effective public decisions.

In fact, efforts to calculate the risks and benefits of technology have often failed to win social acceptability. The fundamental uncertainties about the nature and extent of the risks inherent in many technological choices often defy systematic analysis. Sometimes the effort to quantify risks and benefits masks real technical uncertainties. Moreover, the calculation of risk tends to ignore nonquantifiable, fragile values – the emotional distress or the disruption of social relationships that may be associated with risks. This has led to other lines of inquiry focusing on the factors that enter subjective risk perception.

Beyond the Technical Model

A number of approaches to risk analysis have developed as a reaction to the failure of technical analyses to account for variations in the perception of similar risks in different social, cultural, and institutional contexts. One international comparison of regulatory policies found that:

> The words safe, effective and tolerable are all open to subjective interpretations. Judgments about how many toxic effects are acceptable for a new compound when it enters clinical trials will vary from person to person according to their training and experience, and may also be influenced by their general attitudes towards new chemical substances, chemical manufacturers, or multinational companies [27].

This comparative study suggests that the considerable differences in the assessment and regulation of products to maximize benefits and minimize harm reflect a convergence of medical and political priorities. Irwin [17] and Jasanoff [18] compare national risk policies.

This is the context in which social scientists have entered the "risk business." The earliest set of studies of risk perception focused on individual perceptions and assumed that judgments about risk reflect certain characteristics of the risk itself. A seminal paper by Starr developed several concepts: that risk acceptability increases with increased benefit, and that voluntary risks are more acceptable than involuntary risks [51]. Following up these ideas, psychologists employed laboratory experiments, gaming situations, and survey techniques in order to understand the characteristics of different kinds of risk that seem to influence judgments about their acceptability [13, 14]. Their studies suggest that risks which are involuntary, uncertain, unfamiliar, and potentially catastrophic are most difficult for people to accept. Familiar and voluntary activities, such as smoking, driving, or skiing, may be more dangerous, yet are more easily accepted. Some psychologists extended this list to include other factors such as people's distance from the source of risk and the imaginability of the consequences.

These studies in the field of psychology and decision theory tried to develop a quantitative determination of risk acceptance based on how certain characteristics of the risk itself influence individual perceptions. However, this line of inquiry, limited by its focus on the individual, failed to account for variations in the perception of risk in different social, cultural, and international contexts. Thus the social dimensions of risk perception attracted another line of inquiry among sociologists and anthropologists, who focus on risk as a social or cultural concept [10, 45, 54]. This research, stimulated by the anthropologist Douglas, suggests that concerns about risk may depend less on the nature of the actual danger than on the observer's political, economic, or cultural biases. It is the social system, the ideological premises, and the social tensions within a society that shape perceptions of risk. This is apparent in the concepts of accountability, responsibility, and liability pervading debates about risk and in the fact that such debates frequently include political statements expressing points of tension and value conflicts in a given society.

Sociologists have tended to emphasize the institutional arrangements, social situations, and interests that influence risk perceptions. In the case of pharmaceuticals, for example, consumer calculations are likely to reflect personal health priorities, but the choices are not entirely voluntary. Most lay persons must depend on medical advice, and their evaluations also reflect their personal relationship with a physician and their general trust in professional authority or technical expertise.

In many social situations evaluations of risk become controversial. For example, blue-collar workers are likely to see risks differently than their supervisors. Scientists may view dangers in their laboratories through different lenses than their technicians. Manufacturers interested in marketing products view risks differently than regulators responsible for developing standards to control them [see essays in 40]. Some people talk of risk in terms of cost-effective solutions, of efficiency; others use the language of "rights," emphasizing moral issues and questions of social responsibility, justice, and obligation. Some evaluate risk in statistical terms; others talk of "victims" or "real people." Some define risk as a problem that requires expert solutions; others seek more participatory controls. Such differences imply that research on risk perception must extend beyond narrow questions of health to include the web of social and political issues associated with risk in different social, cultural, or national contexts.

One way to examine the social parameters of risk perception in different cultural contexts is by a comparative study of risk communication. How are risks communicated to the public? What factors influence the dissemination of risk information? How is information assimilated to influence people's attitudes, individual behavior, and public policies? Risk communication is a persistently controversial arena of considerable concern because of its bearing on public perceptions and behavior, on the practices of health professionals, and on regulatory policies. Divergent views on the appropriate way to disseminate information mirror the differences between technical and social approaches to risk that have generally divided the field of risk analysis.

Risk Communication

The mass media are the major but not the only vehicles of risk communication. For the American consumer, newspapers and popular magazines filled with health advisory columns, as well as news about risk events, are the most important source of information. A National Cancer Institute survey of how people become informed about cancer prevention found that 63.6% get their information from magazines, 60% from newspapers, and 58.3% from television. Only 13–15% had talked to their physicians about cancer prevention [37]. Nevertheless, consumers often do seek information from their physicians, as well as from advertising, product labeling and the ubiquitous advisory network that publishes in popular "how-to" books and syndicated health columns. Informal advice from rumors or personal contacts ("my cousin was helped by this drug") also plays an important and often underestimated role in shaping risk perceptions [9].

Health professionals as well as lay persons also use the media as a source of information. Newspaper health columnists report that they receive many inquiries from physicians as well as lay people. But physicians, of course, also have access to scientific research reports and recommendations, to industry's detail men, and to advice from their professional colleagues.

For regulators and public officials the sources of information include scientific research reports and recommendations. However, they are also exposed to information from both industry and consumer advocates who try to influence public policy. Also, regulators rely on the media as an indicator of public opinion.

For many groups in the United States, therefore, the media dominate the avenues of public information. They serve as filters through which people receive news and interpretations of events. Through their coverage or noncoverage of issues they set the agenda of public discourse and affect the priorities guiding personal behavior. The people of the media can move issues to center stage or keep them out of public view. The information that they convey, their visual and verbal images, and the tone of their presentation can define the significance of events, can shape public attitudes, and can legitimate – or call into question – national policies. The timing, content, and tone of media coverage can upset or reassure the public, encouraging complacency or creating fear.

Studies of the media usually focus on the national coverage of specific events [39, 41]. There are few studies comparing media coverage of similar events in different countries. Such studies are particularly difficult. The media operate in given cultural contexts. Their coverage of an issue depends on their political role in a given society, the constraints on public information, the norms and values of the journalistic profession, and the existing views and expectations of their particular audiences. Meaningful cross-national comparisons of the media must consider such variables if they are to illuminate the differences in the coverage of technological risk.

To provide the background for a comparative project I will first draw from the communications literature (mainly in the American context) to suggest how the norms and practices of journalism, the behavior of sources of information, and public expectations shape the reporting of risk. I will then briefly review what is known about the effect of the press in shaping public perceptions and creating policy agendas.

How Do People Know About Risk?

Although the media are diverse even within national contexts[1], they tend to focus on similar kinds of risk issues. Risk events such as accidents or tragedies (e.g., DES

[1] Major newspapers such as the *New York Times* have specialized health and science reporters, ready access to sources of risk information, and other amenities that allow better coverage of the complex issues involved in situations of risk. The smaller daily papers that form the majority of the newspapers in the United States have few specialists and rely heavily on the wire services. Large-circulation weekly magazines have more time to investigate risk issues, but share the competitive constraints of news work that lead to selective focus on dramatic issues. Television communication is especially subject to economic constraints, as well as the demands of visual brevity

daughters or thalidomide) are most newsworthy, especially when they involve human interest stories or personal dramas. So too are dramatic research discoveries that bear on dreaded disease (e. g., potential AIDS therapies or reported "cures" for cancer or Alzheimer's disease). Disputes (e. g., over the safety of birth control pills or swine flu vaccine) are also extensively reported in the press. Less newsworthy is information about routine products or incremental research that might be medically significant but are perceived as neither dramatic nor controversial.

The way in which such issues are reported reflects the organizational constraints of news work: the intense competition, tight deadlines, limited budgets, and the need to cover complex technical subjects within limited space and time. But often the character of media coverage reflects the attitudes of information sources – their tendency toward secrecy or media manipulation and their skill in organizing timely and lucid material for the media. Above all, risk reports in the media reflect the web of social and political issues that are associated with an event. The organization of the media, the behavior of sources of information, and the web of related social and political associations are all likely to differ from country to country, affecting the content and style of the media's coverage of the same event.

Journalists operate under many constraints, including the technical imperatives of news production, economic and editorial pressures, and the perceived need for audience appeal. These constraints are likely to assume quite different configurations in different national contexts. The content and style of reporting, for example, are part of the traditions of journalism, its role in the political system, and the norms and ideologies characteristic of the profession. These are based on patterns and precedents that develop over time. The American press, for example, has been influenced by its origins as a reaction against the excesses of the so-called "yellow journalism" of the nineteenth century and in the early efforts to adapt the norms of scientific objectivity to journalistic practice. Links between the ideals of science and the norms of objective journalism were formed in the mid nineteenth century, when they were perceived as necessary to enhance democratic values and to avoid factionalism in an increasingly diverse and fragmented society [48]. The formation of centralized news syndicates seeking to sell articles to newspaper readers with diverse political views reinforced the role of the media as a cohesive force. Subsequently, in the United States, "objective," that is, unbiased and balanced reporting, has been a journalistic ideal. While newspapers in other countries are tied to political parties or religious groups and are expected to have an explicitly partisan view, American reporters are expected to avoid involvement in political or economic activities that might compromise their neutrality. And they are expected to approach the ideal of objectivity by balancing diverse points of view. Thus journalists cover potentially hazardous technologies or risk events by quoting sources that represent opposing sides of controversial issues, although this gives readers little guidance about the credibility of different views.

The constraints of news work converge with the complexity of technical information about risk to leave most journalists vulnerable to their sources of information. American journalists obtain material for their stories from press releases, conferences, interviews, and selected journals, especially *Science* and the *New England Journal of Medicine (NEJM)*. Those sources best organized to provide technical information to journalists in an efficiently packaged form have a great deal of control over what appears in the press.

In the United States many groups have become highly sophisticated in developing information that has been packaged specifically for the press. Both *Science* and *NEJM* send advance copies to journalists to give them time to write press reports. But because time is short and information complex, most reporters rely heavily on press releases, often adopting their language as well as their content in their news articles.

Approaching the problem of risk communication as a technical issue, industries and scientific groups with interests in controlling perceptions of risk try to provide the "facts" about risk to the media. Corporations have long used scientific and medical images to enhance public confidence in products. But firms are also using scientists themselves in their efforts to manage public perceptions of risk. Public relations firms run so-called "visible scientist" programs for corporate clients, arranging meetings between corporate scientists and editors. They prepare press statements on controversial products and use the credibility of scientists to offset negative publicity about risk [see Chap. 8 in 41]. They have advised corporations to develop "parachute teams" or "truth squads" of scientists to move into risk situations in order to defuse opposition.[2] But such approaches often backfire, becoming a source of cynicism among journalists, who resent the confusion of science with public relations.

Corporations also use the prestige of science as a marketing resource, promoting the benefits of their products by publicizing therapies or products as newsworthy scientific discoveries. But this too can backfire. In 1982 Lilly's arthritis drug, Oraflex, was marketed as "news." The firm's public relations office sent out 6500 press kits promoting this new drug, making scientific claims of its effectiveness. The product was covered as science news by 150 newspapers and television stations, and prescriptions increased from 2000 to 55000 in 1 week. Then a report showed harmful side effects, and the FDA intervened to force the drug off the market. Subsequently the FDA defined such publicity as an extension of drug labeling and tried to control media claims.

Advocacy groups as well as industries perceive the press as a resource through which to mobilize the collective consciousness about risk. A comparative review of environmental policy in the United States, United Kingdom, France, and West Germany found a ubiquitous tendency to use the media as a means to focus political attention on risks [3]. But media relations are likely to differ in part, reflecting national traditions concerning public communication and official secrecy.

If public expectations influence the communication of risk, so too does the web of social and political issues associated with risk. As discussed above, risk is a social concept, and journalistic interpretations reflect attitudes towards authority, the credibility of institutions, and the state of political or economic tensions. The web of social and political issues associated with particular risks influences the way in which they are reported in the press [12].

The issues associated with risks of pharmaceuticals may include economic factors, the availability and cost of health services, the relationship of patients to physicians, and general questions of trust in expertise. Risk may be perceived in terms of the

[2] These phrases are from public relations brochures

reliability of the drug industry, the competence of public health officials, and the effectiveness of government regulation. These social influences on risk perception and communication are a frequent source of conflict. Indeed, risk communication reflects the conflicting social judgments that confound all risk disputes.

First of all, it is seldom clear when best to release information about potential risk to the public. How much evidence is necessary? How certain must the evidence be? How much scientific consensus must there be before research findings are widely reported in the form of news releases or expert recommendations? Views on these questions vary. Most journalists believe that risk data should be promptly available to the public. But some scientists disagree: "Until data are interpreted and validated, until the experimental design and significance are reviewed, and until all currently available data ... can be integrated, the rush to the press is simply mindless, if not unethical [2].[3]

A second set of conflicts over risk communication follows from the different assumptions about how best to communicate risk. Journalistic conventions may violate scientific norms. To create a human interest angle, journalists focus on conflict and create polarities; technologies are either risky or they are safe. Their quest for simplicity, drama, and brevity preclude the nuanced and complex positions that scientists prefer. Moreover, the idea that verity in reporting risk disputes can be established by balancing conflicting claims contradicts the scientists' view that claims must be verified by empirical evidence.

A further set of conflicts follows from the language of risk communication. The very words used to describe risks may have a different meaning in scientific and lay contexts. Biostatisticians use the word "evidence" as a statistical concept. Most lay persons, including journalists, accept anecdotal evidence and individual cases as credible evidence. While scientists talk of aggregate data, reporters write of their readers' immediate concerns: "Will I be harmed?"

Different uses of language can also be found in scientific and policy communications. All groups must summarize and streamline scientific information, selecting particular studies, assigning meaning to particular findings, and deciding the validity of competing claims. A study comparing statements about the link between fiber and colon cancer in reports from the National Academy of Sciences report, the National Cancer Institute, the *NEJM,* and a television documentary found substantial interpretive variations. Although dealing with the same body of information, each report differed on what to emphasize, when to treat a claim as a fact, whether and how to qualify information, and how to deploy the language of uncertainty [16]. The study shows how the social position of actors, their intentions, commitments, and professional interests influenced the communication of policy-relevant science. Indeed, as different groups select, juxtapose, weigh, package, and label evidence, the same corpus of data can assume very different forms.

Such differences may have considerable policy importance. The metaphors and images used to describe a situation can point the finger of blame and imply responsibility for remedial action. Selective use of labels can trivialize an event or render it important; marginalize some groups, empower others; define an issue as an

[3] This philosophy also underlies the "Ingelfinger Rule" that precludes media communication prior to publication in some peer-reviewed journals, in particular the *New England Journal of Medicine*

urgent problem or reduce it to a routine. Was thalidomide a "disaster" or an "incident?" Are chemicals "doomsday products" or "potential risks?" Are risks "normal" and unavoidable, or are they "aberrant" events? Is fear of risk a "phobia" or simply a "concern?"

The choice of language, as a reflection of values, is also strategic, for language carries implications for the formulation of policy. For example, defining the problems of risk in terms of insufficient technical evidence implies that "risk assessment," with its connotations of objectivity, is the appropriate approach to regulation, and that regulation is properly the province of expertise. Defining the problems in the social or moral context of responsibility and social justice, on the other hand, calls for more political approaches to public policy. In this way, the discourse frames both risk perceptions and the policy agenda [40].

The Influence of Risk Communication

Some insight into the influence of risk communication can be gained from studies of media effects on public attitudes (review: 35]. Some studies stress the media's pervasive influence in shaping our values, habits, and ideals [see e. g. 15]. Others view the media communication of risk as a kind of narcosis. "The avalanche of popular articles dealing with the possible risks associated with the use or nonuse of various foods, drugs, chemicals and energy systems may well be calculated not to help in the making of wise choices, but rather to prevent the making of any choices at all" [44, 55]. Most research has found a somewhat limited influence. The media's primary effect has been aptly described as "agenda setting." "The press may not be successful much of the time in telling people what to think, but it is stunningly successful in telling its readers what to think about" [34].

Research also indicates that increased technical information may have relatively little influence on public reactions to risk. If people's responses depended on instrumental cost-benefit calculations, then knowledge would clearly enhance enlightened choice. But responses to risk tend to coincide with political values and general faith in technology. People are, according to one study, influenced more by their peers and social contacts than by their knowledge of technical details [25]. One study of the media coverage of nuclear power found little evidence of media influence. Despite the perceptions of the nuclear power industry, which tended to blame the press for many of its ills, the study concluded that "the press ... is honored more as a talking point than an action force; and judged more puissant by those it criticizes than would be merited by its actions" [11]. Another study suggests that the quantity of coverage of a risk event may have more influence on public perceptions than the content of the coverage [33].

The general thrust of communication research suggests that information is assimilated and interpreted in different ways, depending on prior beliefs, predispositions, personal experience, and the attitudes of peers; that media communication is but a contributing factor to, not the primary cause of, the public's attitudes and ideas [1, 23, 29]. The effect of risk information, then, is likely to depend on the social and cultural context, as well as the particular social situation in which it is received. Especially important are the attitudes held by opinion leaders in a given community. The social context includes the educational background and expectations of readers, as well as their alternative sources of information and imagery, such as television programs, comic strips, and other vehicles of popular culture.

The influence of risk information on attitudes is also likely to vary with the selective interest and personal experience of the receiver. In "esoteric" areas, where newspaper readers or television viewers have little direct information or preexisting knowledge to guide an independent evaluation (e.g., the effect of fluorocarbons on the ozone in the atmosphere), the media was found to be the major source of information. In effect, the media defined the reality of the situation and played a critical role in shaping perceptions of the risk [8]. In contrast, where readers already have an established set of biases or long-term exposure to press coverage (as in the case of reporting about certain environmental issues), media reports tend to justify and reinforce existing views. And when a person has had personal experience (e.g., with workplace risks or with particular medications), the influence of media images on risk perception is tempered by prior attitudes [30, 50].

The influence of risk information on actual behavior (e.g., consumer choices) depends on a number of variables. Reports about risk are most likely to affect consumer behavior if alternative products are available. News coverage of toxic shock syndrome adversely affected the sales of some brands of tampons. After extensive media reports on dietary studies relating cholesterol-producing foods to heart disease, consumption of beef, eggs, and fatty milk products declined. Similarly, reports on the risks of excessive sodium consumption increased the use of salt-free food products [43].

Publicity about the possible adverse effects of birth control pills and IUDs also resulted in a significant decline in their use. This decline, between 1970 and 1975, correlated directly with the press coverage of Congressional hearings on birth control methods, the studies linking the use of contraceptive pills to the risk of strokes, and the FDA warning to women over 40 about the increased risk of heart attacks among those using the pill. Each news disclosure brought sharp changes in behavior [20].

A number of factors are likely to affect consumer behavior in response to risk information about pharmaceutical products. Persons deciding whether or not to use a drug must trade off the risks of an adverse drug response against the benefits to be gained. The decision may rest on personal attitudes towards comfort or pain, on trust in health professionals, or on the manner in which health advice was provided. It may also depend on their sense of control over their situation and their belief in traditional folk wisdom about health and disease. Similarly, risk information is likely to affect the activities of consumer groups in ways that reflect social factors such as their confidence in regulatory authorities and trust in the integrity of industrial producers of pharmaceutical products.

Deliberate efforts to use the press to influence behavior do not necessarily have the effect anticipated. Despite extensive news coverage of the Salk polio vaccine when it became available in the late 1950s, relatively few individuals agreed to be vaccinated at that time [46]. Similarly, media coverage of the 1964 Surgeon General's report on smoking and cancer had little apparent direct effect on smoking habits in the short term [56]. Although people seek risk information from the media to guide even the most personal decisions (such as choice of birth control techniques), they actually use such information mainly when it corresponds to their prior inclinations.

A more general effect of media coverage is to establish a framework of expectations, so that isolated events take on meaning as public issues [57]. The media, in effect, make problems visible and define a "frame" or context in which related events can be interpreted. In this way media reports set the public agenda and influence policy decisions.

By their selection of newsworthy events journalists identify pressing policy issues. By their focus on controversial issues they stimulate demands for accountability, forcing policy makers to justify themselves to a larger public [26]. By their use of images they help to create the judgmental biases that underlie public policy. The importance of this last tool must not be underestimated. The real power of the press, claimed Laski, comes from "its ability to surround facts by an environment of suggestions which, often half consciously, seeks its way into the mind of the reader and forms his premises for him" [28]. Metaphors in science journalism cluster and reinforce one another, creating consistent, coherent, and therefore powerful images which often have strategic policy implications. When technology is associated with "frontiers" that are maintained through "battles" or "struggles," the imagery of war implies that the experts should not be questioned, that new technologies must go forward, and that limits are inappropriate. But if, instead, the imagery suggests peril, crisis, or technology out of control, we seek ways to "rein in" the runaway forces through increased government regulation and control.

The policy influence of risk communication is apparent in many areas. It was the media coverage of the controversy over recombinant DNA research that led the mayor of Cambridge, Massachusetts to organize a citizens' review board to evaluate the wisdom of building a laboratory in the city [24]. News publicity surrounding the debate over Laetrile as a cancer cure forced the National Cancer Institute to test the drug on human cancer patients even though the lack of therapeutic effects on animals normally would have precluded human testing [32].

By creating public issues out of events, the press can force regulatory agencies to action simply out of concern for their public image. Within 4 days of the initial press reports on experiments finding bladder malignancy in rats exposed to high doses of cyclamates, the commissioner of the Food and Drug Administration put in place the cyclamate ban. This was perhaps a record for the rapidity of an administrative response to a technical study. Why such haste on the basis of limited evidence? "We were afraid of a leak," said the commissioner. He feared that public exposure in the press would politicize the FDA's activities and bring about legislative oversight [5].

Press coverage can also influence the financial support given to research, a fact well understood by scientists and their institutions. In the 1940s the proliferation of cancer stories in the press helped to convince Congress to give research support to the National Cancer Institute. The dramatization of infantile paralysis in the press in the 1950s attracted millions of dollars to the support of research in this area. More recently, dramatic news stories about AIDS generated public funds for AIDS research, and media pressure forced the release of AZT (azidothymidine) as a therapy for AIDS before the completion of controlled clinical trials.

Evidence of media influence has encouraged a ubiquitous tendency to "blame the messenger" for problems associated with risk and has spawned proposals to limit media access to information. Both industry and government agencies have reasons to restrict public communication about risk. Public discussion of potential risks could lead to the intrusion of burdensome regulations, fuel compensation claims, or require the installation of costly equipment to reduce risks. Disclosure of data about safety could also erode the ability of companies to reap the economic benefits of their work by interfering with industrial trade secrecy [53].

Sometimes it is feared that the difficulties of communicating the details of technical problems and conveying the significance of statements of probability will result in hasty and inappropriate public responses. Thus, in various countries questions are raised about the wisdom of disclosure. Are there times when nondisclosure of risk might be desirable? Should the media suppress information because of its potential impact? The response is likely to vary according to national expectations. The American public, for example, expects to be informed. There have been efforts to limit media access to sensitive risk information (e.g., the exclusion of reporters from the Asilomar conference on the risks of recombinant DNA) and attempts to discourage scientists from talking directly to reporters by setting up professional liaisons responsible for distilling information for the press. However, such constraints are invariably controversial. Expectations are quite different in countries with varying levels of central control over the media and different traditions of official secrecy [18, 42].

Clearly there are dangers in disclosing information about potential risks; the cost of public scrutiny may be high, and complex issues can be trivialized in the course of public debate. To call public attention to uncertainty even in the most even-handed way is to challenge professional competence and control. To raise questions about the sources of risk is to challenge the authority and legitimacy of decision-making procedures. And to publicize a problem of risk is to take it beyond consideration by experts to the arena of public debate. But in all countries these costs must be weighed against the imperatives of open communication. Despite the difficulties of media communication about controversial technological issues and the cost of public scrutiny, there remain sound political, ethical and pragmatic reasons for improving media access to risk information. Information is a political resource.

In the United States context, it is widely believed that media access to information about the risks as well as the benefits of technology is central to the existence of an informed citizenry able to engage knowledgeably in political choices. A National Academy of Sciences committee has claimed that the dissemination of information about risks is an ethical imperative, based on "the concern of society as a whole with the individual's right of self-determination" [36]. Right-to-know laws and federal regulations about disclosure of product contents in consumer goods are based on the principle that informed consent must take precedence over efficiency.

Timely communication of information on risks to the public may also have practical importance. Media coverage may exaggerate the problem of risks, but by increasing public awareness it may also elicit the support that is necessary to bring risks under control. It may force public officials to be accountable to their constituents. And it may help bring critical problems to the policy agenda.

There is also evidence that information about the risks as well as the benefits of science and technology may have strong bearing on institutional credibility and the public's trust [60]. The risks of advancing technologies have contributed to an erosion of belief in the value of science and technology as instruments of progress and to a decline of public confidence in the legitimacy of decision-making institutions.

Neither the problem of technological risk nor concerns about risk communication are new issues, but they have assumed new dimensions in many countries. The problem of risk has been magnified by the increasing dangers brought about by new technologies. The impact of the media has been magnified by changes in communication capacity and scale. Understanding the forces that shape the perception and communication of risk in an international context is thus increasingly important to the efforts to define and implement acceptable policies for technological change.

A Proposed Research Agenda

I offer this proposal as a set of guidelines for an international project that would systematically compare the communication of similar risk issues in different countries. Focusing on the risks and benefits of pharmaceutical products and following the material presented in this background paper, the project would address several questions:
- What means of risk communication are employed in different national contexts, and how do various groups obtain information that would help them weigh risks and benefits?
- How are communication practices shaped by national differences, e.g., in the organization of the media, expectations about public knowledge, and the interests and activities of various sources of information?
- What is the influence of risk communication on attitudes, behavior, and public policy, and what social factors affect the way in which information is assimilated?

To implement this proposal scholars from different countries who are familiar with the media would be commissioned to write papers on these questions as they related to a shared issue. To facilitate comparison, each paper would follow the same outline dealing with the same questions. The project could include three types of risk issues:
- Accidents or dramatic events.
- Research discoveries.
- Disputes over potentially hazardous products.

Each study would address the same problem and in each case would examine the following questions.

The diverse channels of risk and benefit communication:
1. The role of advertising, detail men, and other industry-generated sources.
2. Government reports from both scientific and policy groups.
3. The role of advocacy or community health groups in communicating risks and benefits.
4. The media.

The national context of risk communication:
1. Organization of the media, including material on historically based norms, political linkages, anticipated readership, distribution patterns of different types of media, and government control over the media.

2. The sources of information, including material on norms of openness versus secrecy, the use of media by interest groups, what journalists use for sources, and how various groups influence journalists.
3. The issue webs, that is, the social and political questions associated with the risk, including national experience with similar problems, the nature of the health care system, and practices and expectations about regulation.

Media coverage patterns, including:
1. Amount of coverage of a risk issue, its placement in the press, the timing of coverage, and the length of time that media interest in the issue is sustained.
2. Decisions about nondisclosure. What is covered in some countries and not in others?
3. Characteristics of the coverage, including key and repeated metaphors and images, the level of technical detail, the statements of public officials or well-known figures, the sources that are cited as experts (industry, government, and advocacy groups), the notions of balance and responsibility, and the definition of the stakes that are involved.

Influence of communication:
1. Survey research to indicate (a) influence of communication on attitudes and behavior and (b) questions of trust and credibility.
2. Analysis of documents (court proceedings, hearings).
3. Indicators of the effect of communication on regulatory policies (e.g., on setting of standards).
4. Social experiments that would utilize focus groups to assess the effects of communication about risks and benefits. A model exists in the media round tables in which risk reporters participate in seminars with scientists. The effect on their reporting could then be evaluated.

The commissioned papers would be presented at a conference or series of working sessions directed towards developing a book. The conference chairperson would be responsible for editing and coordinating the volume and writing an introductory analytic essay.

References

1. Bauer R, Bauer A (1960) America, mass society and mass media. J. Social Issues 16: 3–66
2. Bloom B (1979) News about carcinogens; what is fit to print. Hastings Center Report, August: 5–7
3. Brickman R, Jasanoff S, Ilgen T (1985) Controlling chemicals: the politics of regulation in Europe and the U.S. Cornell University Press, Ithaca, NY
4. Clark University Decision Research Project (1979) Project summary: improving the societal management of technological hazards Clark University, Eugene, Oregon
5. Cooper J (1970) Cyclamate sequel: risks dominating benefits. Med Tribune, 26 February: 11
6. Covello V, Abernathy M (1983) Risk analysis and technological hazards: a policy-related bibliography. In: Whipple C et al. (eds) Technological risk assessment. Sijthoff and Nordhoff, Amsterdam
7. Crandall RC (1977) Curbing the cost of social regulation. Brookings Bull 15: 1–15

8. Dotto L, Schiff H (1978) The ozone war. Doubleday, New York, chap 7
9. Douglas M (1985) Risk acceptability according to the social sciences. Russell Sage Foundation, New York, pp 70–71
10. Douglas M, Wildavsky A (1982) Risk and culture. University of California, Berkeley
11. Eisendruth C, Broder J (1979) The media connection. In: Schramm G (ed) The value of time. School of Natural Resources, Ann Arbor
12. Enloe C (1975) The politics of pollution in a comparative perspective. McKay, New York
13. Fischoff B, Slovic P, Lichtenstein S (1979) Which risks are acceptable? Environment 21: 17–38
14. Fischoff B, Lichtenstein S, Slovic P, Derby S, Keeney R (1981) Acceptable risk. Cambridge University Press, New York
15. Gans H (1979) Deciding what's news. Pantheon, New York
16. Hilgartner S (1988) The diet and cancer debate, chap 9 of PhD thesis. Cornell University
17. Irwin A (1985) Risk and the control of technology. Manchester University Press
18. Jasanoff S (1986) Risk management and political culture. Russell Sage Foundation, New York
19. Jasanoff S (1987) Unscrambling the messages on risk, Sci Technol Human Values, October
20. Jones E et al. (1980) Pill and IUD discontinuation in the US 1970–1975; influence of the media. Family Planning Perspectives 12: 293–300
21. Kates RW (1979) Risk assessment of environmental hazards. Wiley, New York
22. Kates RW, Hohenemser C (eds) (1981) Technological hazard management. Oelgeshlagger, Gunn & Hain, Cambridge MA
23. Klapper J (1960) The effects of mass communication. The Free Press, Glencoe
24. Krimsky S (1983) Genetic alchemy. MIT Press, Cambridge
25. Kuhlinski J et al. (1982) Citizen knowledge and choices on the complex issue of nuclear energy. Am J Polit Sci, November
26. Lang G, Lang K (1983) The battle for public opinion. Columbia University Press, New York
27. Lasagna L, Werkö L (1986) International differences in drug regulation philosophy. Int J Technol Assess Health Care 2: 616
28. Laski H (1984) The american democracy. Viking Press, New York
29. Lazarsfeld P et al. (1944) The people's choice. Duell, Sloan and Pierce, New York
30. Lemert J (1981) Does press communication change public opinion after all? Nelson Hall, Chicago, pp 44–45
31. Majone G (1977) Standard setting and a theory of institutional choice. Policy and Politics 5
32. Markle G (1982)The politics of Laetrile. Sage, Beverly Hills
33. Mazur A (1987) The dynamics of technological controversy. Communications Press, Washington DC
34. McCombs ME, Shaw DL (1972) The agenda-setting role of the mass media. Public Opinion 36: 176
35. McQuail D (1979) The influence and effects of mass media. In: Curran J et al. (eds) Mass communication and society. Sage, Beverly Hills (chap 3)
36. National Research Council, National Academy of Sciences (1978) Informing workers and employers about cancer. U.S. Government Printing Office, Washington DC, p 5
37. National Cancer Institute (1984) Cancer prevention awareness survey. U.S. Government Printing Office, Washington DC, pp 58, 64 (NIH report 84-26-77)
38. Nelkin D (ed) (1984) Controversy: the politics of technical decisions, 2nd edn. Sage, Beverly Hills
39. Nelkin D (1984) Background paper for Twentieth Century Fund (ed) Science in the streets: the communication of technical risk. Priority Press, New York
40. Nelkin D (ed) (1985) The language of risk. Sage, Beverly Hills
41. Nelkin D (1987) Selling science: how the press covers science and technology. Freeman, New York
42. Nelkin D, Pollak M (1981) The pregnant pause: the European response to Three Mile Island. In: Moss T, Sills D (eds) The Three Mile Island nuclear accident. New York Academy of Sciences, New York
43. New York Times, December 9, 1984 and October 19, 1985
44. Postman N (1980) News as narcosis. The Nation, 1 March: 4–5
45. Rayner S (1984) Disagreeing about risk. In: Hadley SG (ed) Risk analysis, institutions and public policy. Associated Faculty Press, Port Washington, NY
46. Robinson EJ (1963) Analyzing the impact of science reporting. Journalism Q 40: 306–314

47. Rowe W (1977) An anatomy of risk. Wiley, New York
48. Schiller D (1981) Objectivity and the news. University of Pennsylvania Press, Philadelphia
49. Schwartz RC, Alberts WA (eds) (1980) How safe is safe enough? Plenum, New York
50. Seymour-Ure C (1968) The press, politics and the public. Methuen, London
51. Starr C (1969) Social benefit vs. technological risk. Science, 19 September: 1232–1238
52. Starr C, Whipple C (1980) The risk of risk decision. Science, 6 June: 1114
53. Stevenson R Jr (1980) Corporations and information. Johns Hopkins University Press, Baltimore
54. Thompson M (1982) A proposal to create a cultural theory of risk. In: Kunreuther H, Ley E (eds) The risk analysis controversy Springer, Berlin Heidelberg New York
55. Trachman L (1981) The public understanding of science effort. Sci Technol Human Values, summer: 13
56. Troyer R, Markle G (1983) Cigarettes. Rutgers University Press, New Brunswick
57. Tuchman G (1978) Making news. Free Press, New York
58. Tversky A, Kahnemann D (1974) Judgment under uncertainty. Science 185: 1124–1131
59. U.S. Department of Health and Human Services (1986) Determining risk to health: federal policy and practice. Auburn House
60. Yankelovich D (1982) Changing public attitudes to science and the quality of life. Sci Technol Human Values 39: 23–29

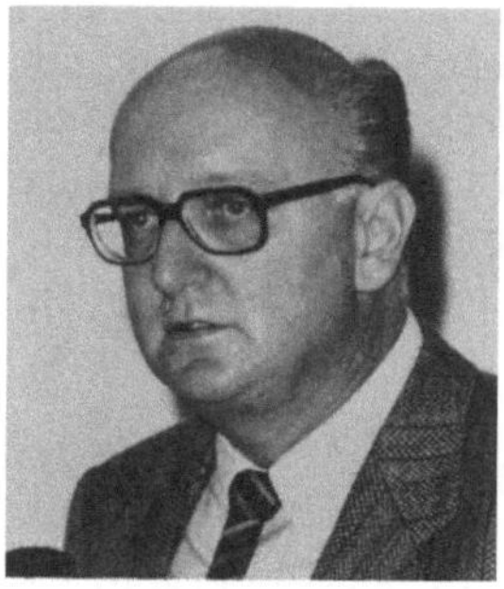

4. Overview of the Drug Safety Issue and Ciba-Geigy's Response: RAD-AR

W. P. von Wartburg

Introduction

I would like to open my presentation on the Ciba-Geigy programme of "Risk Assessment of Drugs – Analysis and Response" (RAD-AR) by answering some questions that may be uppermost in your minds: Why are we here? What are the objectives of the conference? Let me observe two things here.

The first objective is collectively to improve our knowledge in terms of having a state-of-the-art practice in dealing with drug side-effects. Each of the companies represented here has very specialized knowledge in very specialized fields. If we can somehow exchange this expertise, I think that we will all benefit from each other. I would encourage you to be quite open and frank in your exchange of experience. The first objective is thus to improve the state of the art in dealing with adverse drug reactions.

The second, and perhaps more important, objective is to encourage industry cooperation in various specific projects. We hope that by the end of this conference there will be sufficient interest from some of you to allow us to move forward in a collaborative way. A number of projects will be presented with this objective in mind.

Now, you may ask, does this represent same kind of "collusion" behaviour? The answer is "no". We will not be discussing anything which could affect competition. We may be discussing company-specific issues, but only in the broader context of their implications for optimizing the safety of drugs in the interest of patients. If together we are able to come to certain conclusions which can benefit the patient by improving the state of the art, this has nothing to do with anti-competitive behaviour.

Another question that you may have is: "If this is an industry-wide issue, why is the meeting being held by Ciba-Geigy rather than by an industry association?" The answer is that our industry associations represent the interests of all members, large or small, research-based or not, across a wide variety of issues. We debated among ourselves and concluded that it made more sense to invite those companies with similar operations (research-based, international activities) and similar experiences. But we certainly did not want to exclude the industry associations, and I am pleased that representatives of IFPMA are participating in this conference.

This is not a closed or secretive meeting. To demonstrate this, we have invited representatives of the media. We do not have anything to hide, and we want an open exchange of views.

And, of course, we also welcome independent experts from the various disciplines related to the issues under discussion. How were these chosen? In developing our RAD-AR programme, we took many soundings, did our own research, and hope that we have chosen outstanding representatives in the respective disciplines. They are certainly all of independent minds and are under no commitment whatsoever to report what we might want them to report.

Looking Back 100 Years

I find it interesting to reflect on life some 100 years ago. Around 1885–1890 gold was discovered in South Africa; golf was introduced to America; in England, the Lawn Tennis Association was founded; Jack the Ripper was murdering in London; and New York and Vienna were about the same size, namely one million inhabitants. We also had a global influenza epidemic which was frightening at the time.

How did science and technology look 100 years ago? The Canadian Pacific Railway had just been completed; the underground was opened in London; the steam engine turbine was invented; Karl Benz built the first motorcar engine; George Eastman of Kodak manufactured photographic paper; and John Dunlop invented the pneumatic tyre.

One hundred years ago there were also notable drug innovations. Phenacetin was discovered, as was tetanus bacillus; Louis Pasteur devised a rabies vaccine; aminopyrine (which recently became very much a drug issue) was developed, as was insulin.

Ten Years Ago

No one here remembers the world of 100 years ago because none of you were around at that time, but you all probably remember 10 years ago. And what was happening then? I begin again with some interesting facts about daily life. The unemployment rate in the United States was over 9%; London suffered its worst underground crash; the British pound and the Italian lira were at all-time low levels against the United States dollar; Legionnaires' disease was rampant; 800000 people died in earthquakes; and on the shores of Brittany the Amoco Cadiz was breaking apart.

In terms of science and technology, let me give, again, just a few highlights. It was roughly 10 years ago that we had the first reports on potential ozone layer depletion damage. We had the first manned space shuttle; we had the first testing of the neutron bomb. And regarding tests, we had the first test-tube baby born in England. Ten years ago saw the first construction of a functional synthetic gene at the Massachusetts Institute of Technology. This is more or less the climate which was to shape the present.

In terms of drug innovation, the first successful treatment of herpes encephalitis took place 10 years ago. Cimetidine was around the corner for the treatment of gastric ulcers; captopril became available for combatting hypertension; and human calcitonine was put into use against Paget's disease.

Today's Anxieties

Out of the climate of problems and developments in recent years have grown today's anxieties. Reducing these to the lowest common denominator, we see that most are concerned in one way or another with environmental pollution – radiation hazards, pesticides and acid-rain – to name but a few.

Drug risks also constitute a major anxiety today. This drug risk issue in cultural or historical terms is an outgrowth of what we have seen in recent years. What has happened during this time?

If we look only at the 1980s, we see a phenomenon which was and still is difficult to explain. A number of old, established drugs have suddenly disappeared. We find quite a number of newly introduced "wonder" drugs being withdrawn after a promising start. The number of drug issues has been rising rather dramatically. And both manufacturers and drug-regulatory authorities have come under increasing public criticism.

Reasons for Drug Criticism

A great number of drugs has been severely restricted or is no longer available. Looking only at individual cases, this is perhaps not so striking, but if one regards the whole range of drugs which have disappeared, there must be some reasons, some common factors. There certainly have been reasons with respect to activities or non-activities by the companies involved and the adverse drug reaction profiles of their products. But there have also been reasons outside the company, beyond the control of the company, involving communication, and having to do with perceptions. And it is on these issues that I hope we can dwell in some detail at this conference. I would like quickly to list these for you.

Looking at the reasons for drug criticism which in the end leads to the disappearance of drugs, simplifying, one can say that it has either been a question of lack of efficacy, of poor quality, of inappropriate information, of insufficient cost-effectiveness or of safety problems (Fig. 4.1). I would like to go quickly through each of these and illustrate what I mean.

When efficacy is the issue, clearly the drug does not work. Perhaps the indications are not sufficiently proven; there may be a lack of clinical trials in the relevant patient populations, doubtful clinical end points, bad trial times and so on. These are some of the efficacy issues which can lead to criticism and the disappearance of a drug.

But there are also issues of quality, such as substandard manufacturing practices and lack of consistent quality. This represents a classic case of a recall if the drug is defective.

Then there is the issue of information: if information is not balanced, if warning statements or contraindications are lacking, if there is excessive promotion – in other words, if the drug information is not correct or is misleading – disappearance of the drug may result.

The next issue I would like to outline is that of cost-effectiveness: a drug which does not represent good value for money can also attract severe criticism. If the cost-benefit relationship is not balanced, if the price is not in relation to the medical value,

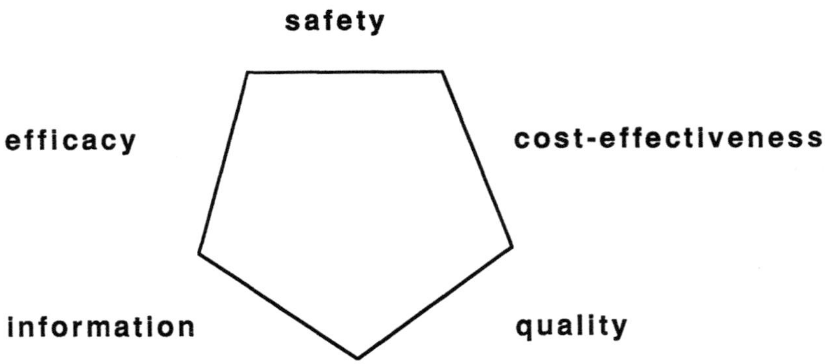

Efficacy Issues

- Indications not sufficiently proven
- Lack of clinical trials in relevant patient populations
- Doubtful clinical endpoints
- Bad trial designs or inappropriate measurements or parameters

= drug does not work

Safety Issues

- Too many side effects
- Too severe side effects
- Treatment risk inappropriately high
- Comparative benefit/risk relationship doubtful

= drug does not have a positive benefit/risk relationship

Cost-effectiveness Issues

- Excessive pricing
- Cost-benefit relation not balanced
- Price not in relation to medical value
- Improvement of quality of life questionable

= drug does not represent good value for money

Information/Promotion Issues

- Indications are not backed up by sufficient clinical data
- Information is not balanced
- Warning statements/contraindications are lacking
- Promotion is excessive

= drug information is incorrect

Quality Issues

- Substandard manufacturing practices
- Lack of consistent quality
- Insufficient quality control

= drug is defective

Fig. 4.1. The pentagram of drug criticism

or if improvement of quality of life is questionable, substantial criticism may be levelled at a drug and may have an impact on the life of the drug.

But where we really come to the crux of the issue is in the area of safety. It is obvious that there must be efficacy, quality, information and cost-effectiveness, but one must also demonstrate safety. Safety issues are characterized by too many side-effects, too severe side-effects, inappropriately high treatment risk, or doubtful comparative benefit-risk relationship. In other words, if the drug does not have a positive, demonstrable benefit-risk relationship, it may well have a short-lived future.

Can We Predict Future Drug Issues?

These have probably been the most prominent reasons for the disappearance of drugs, both old and new. And when we look a little into the future, we must recognize that which is being criticized in 1988 may become a big issue in 1989. The question arises as to whether we can, to some extent, forecast the future. I would now like to present a model that we have developed which deals with what I call the awareness life-cycle of drug risk-benefit issues.

Drug issues usually begin within the company. Concerns then somehow show up in scientific/medical circles. Here they are still within the family, so to speak, because the issue is contained within the medical establishment. But when these reports enter the professional press, suddenly there is public media coverage. With public media coverage comes consumer interest, and with consumer interest comes political pressure. As a result of political pressure there is sometimes administrative action, in some cases leading to restrictions, withdrawal, or the cancellation of a drug licence. We have tried to look at all drug issues which have been raised in the professional press. We cannot catch all questions within all companies, nor can we catch everything which is said in scientific and medical circles. But we can catch an issue when it is raised in the professional press, such as *Scrip, Health Action International, Arzneimitteltelegramm, Drug Letter* and similar publications. These are the professional reports which most likely will lead to coverage by the public media and enter the kind of interest cycle that I have described.

Over a period of 15 months we screened these journals to ascertain the kind of drug issues reported there and noted whether the reports concerned efficacy, quality, information, cost-effectiveness or safety. We then put this information into a data base with a programme which identified the drug, the manufacturer, the event which led to the criticism, the critics and the source of reporting.

We found that between January 1987 and the end of March 1988, there were 617 drug issues. Of these, some 130 were related to efficacy, 23 to quality, and some 100 to information. Not surprisingly, almost 500 out of the 617 events monitored concerned safety. This confirms, in my view, that the safety issue is at the forefront of public thought, and that we will have to deal increasingly with this issue in future.

As with all such programmes, we can conduct subset analyses. We can discover whether drug safety issues are more preponderant in one class of drugs than another, whether issues arise more in one country than another, which companies have been affected and to what degree, and so on.

To the extent that drug safety issues move from the professional press into the lay media and hence into the public and political arena, such a model helps us to monitor trends and forecast future issues.

The Risk-Benefit Relationship

We now come to the issues intended for more detailed discussion in the 2 days to come. Drug risks must be seen in the context of corresponding benefits. These benefits should not be seen merely in a medical but also in a social and economic light. We have always proved medical benefits; we can demonstrate clinical evidence related to quality of life, the cost-benefit relationship and cost-effectiveness so that these social and economic data can be put into context with the risks which we also see in pharmaceuticals.

Lowrance has presented at this conference a "triad" of assessment, appraisal and response. Interestingly, I came up with something similar, namely analysis, appraisal and management. I feel that, like any other health hazard, drug risks need first to be analysed, then appraised and then managed. All three elements of analysis, appraisal and management involve not only scientific and factual elements but also societal and political value judgements. They require state-of-the-art knowledge and state-of-the-art behaviour. This applies to public health risks in general as well as to drug risks.

The additional elements which enter here are perception and communication. These play an increasingly important role, and we will talk about them as well. Let me just run quickly through risk analysis and some of the things which ought to be done.

First, and obvious to you as experts, we must improve reporting on adverse drug reactions and standardize some of the prevalence and incidence calculations. This is not yet done in a satisfactory way. We must then assure sound probability assessments. We also need to strengthen our in-house pharmaco-epidemiology systems because I think this can better provide answers in dealing with the epidemiological background of a drug and with risks which are often seen out of context.

As regards appraisal, we should evaluate much more the seriousness of drug risks on a comparative basis. This does not mean attempting a kind of negative marketing on the basis of side effects but finding out what it really means to the patient if one drug is no longer prescribed while another one is. We should judge the severity of the risk in relation to the effects of the untreated disease. We should make our value judgements about acceptable risks explicit and should not be ashamed of doing so. And we should always try to balance these risks against the corresponding benefits of a medical, social or economic nature.

One way of managing drug risk is by improving information. This cannot be repeated too often. We should also try to fine-tune the intensity of intervention on our part to the relative degree of risk. We should ensure post-marketing surveillance with fast follow-up. If we obtain new results, we must make sure that we also act quickly, that we do not merely have the results somewhere on file. And we should do substantial pharmaco-epidemiological monitoring of the benefit-risk relationship during the whole lifetime of a drug.

Reality, Perception and Communication

Now, let me come briefly to the issues of perception and communication. I think all these three elements, analysis, appraisal and management, have to do not only with facts or realities but also with perceptions. And perceptions are something which can be changed by communication, and which are interrelated with our communication behaviour. Perceptions are important because they deal with perceived realities. And human action is motivated as much by perception as it is by reality.

Communication is essential for the purpose of providing facts, changing perceptions (where this is needed) and transferring convictions from one partner to the other. Nothing speaks for itself in the area of drug risk analysis, appraisal and management. For long we in the pharmaceutical industry have believed certain things to be self-explanatory. They were all too obvious – so why talk about them? And thus we remained passive and silent. But they are not self-explanatory; they have simply been misunderstood. I am convinced that effective communication is the key to the handling of risks and also to risk acceptance by society.

It is evident that in the area of drug risks, reality and perceived reality can differ. If perceptions about drug risks are formed on the basis of what people know, hear, read or see, people will judge drug risks on their personal experience. If drug risks in a given instance are perceived by a majority of the public as being unacceptable, then a new reality exists which may take precedence over established scientific and medical facts. And there is absolutely no need for a lament afterwards by the scientists who say "but this is not so". If it is *perceived* as being so, it effectively *is* the reality.

This is something which, especially within medical and scientific circles, is almost unheard of because we cling to pharmacological and toxicological data, and these represent truth to us; they are our reality. But in the context of public opinion there are different realities, perceived realities. And if these become the majority, based among the public, they take precedence over the "real" reality. Drug regulatory authorities, which are in effect political bodies simply cannot disregard such perceived realities.

What does this mean in terms of communication? We must move from the "old" publics to the "new" publics and from the "old" language to the "new" language (Table 4.1). This is the key message. If we concentrate on our old publics with our old, established language, I do not think we are going to improve anywhere. We must also move from what I would describe as "old behaviour" to "new behaviour". The old behaviour was reactive rather than proactive, selective rather than collective, information-based rather than communication-based, and consisted of a monologue rather than a dialogue. We should not be afraid to participate in public debate and, indeed,

Table 4.1. Drug risk communication: past and future

Past	Future
Old publics	*New publics*
Medical professions	Patients
Scientific communities	Public at large
Regulatory authorities	Politicians
	Media representatives
	Consumer organizations
	Special interest groups
Old language	*New language*
Medical/scientific	Patient-oriented
Restricted, expert wording	Commonly understandable terms
Old behaviour	*New behaviour*
Preactive	Proactive
Selective	Collective
Information	Communication
Monologue	Dialogue
Old contents	*New contents*
Image campaigns	Management of existing perceptions
	Management of prevailing anxieties

should help set the agenda for debate. This means speaking out when necessary with clear, consistent messages.

We should also move from image-based campaigns which benefit primarily advertising agencies to the management of existing perceptions and the management of prevailing anxieties. To do this we need perception analysis, for we need to know much more about how the public feels and what patients themselves experience. We must also go out and discover these perceptions so that we can manage them effectively. Trust cannot be bought, it must be earned by openness, by state-of-the-art policies and by state-of-the-art activities.

5. Summary of Part I: Presentations and Discussions

The first speakers focused on the importance of evaluating risks, in general, and health risks, in particular. They traced how man has taken both known and unknown risks in order to find new options and to make progress both in culture and technology. They observed that a society which only considers safety in the face of risk would cease to develop, and innovation would be hindered if not halted. By weighing risk against benefits, we have created and employed the concept of "acceptable risk."

Nothing in life – including pharmaceuticals – is without risk; one must constantly choose between risk and benefit. From the beginning, one learns to *assess, appraise,* and *respond to* or *manage* each risk. The assessment should survey a scope of considerations, including personal, technological, social, and economic.

During the past 10 years, we have witnessed increasing interest in risk assessment and perception. Differences in the *perception* of risk are partially a function of the different social, cultural, and international contexts in which they occur. Understand-

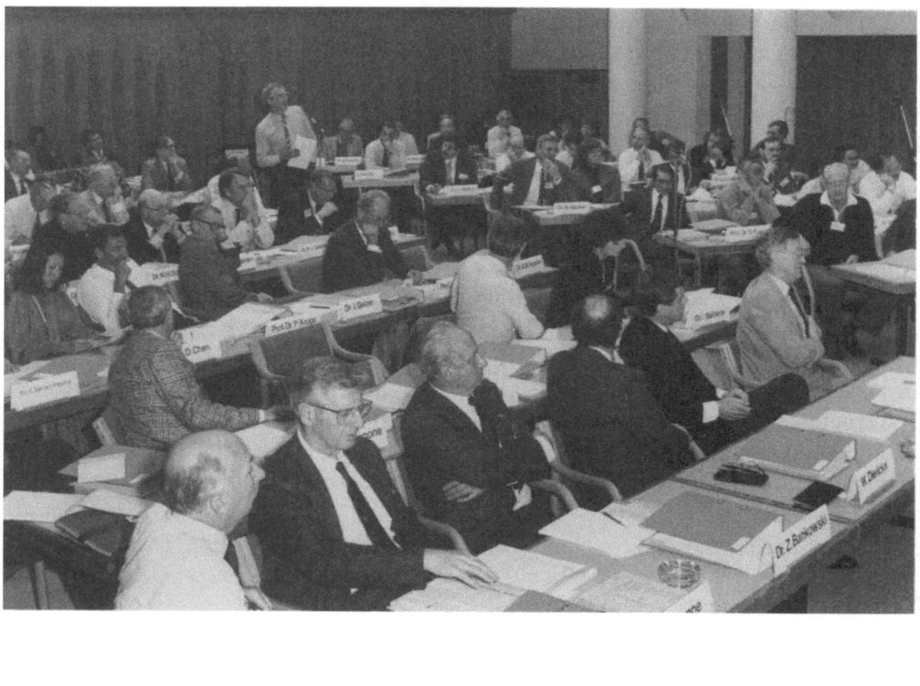

ing the forces which shape the perception and communication of risk has become increasingly important in order to define and implement policies for technological change. For instance, concerns about risk may depend less on actual danger than on the biases of the observer.

Risk may be defined as a probability of harm coupled with its magnitude or consequence. Risk-response actions may be viewed as investments, actions that return something to a person or society. It is, of course, unwise to make an investment without good indications that the benefits will outweigh the negative effects.

Our agenda concerning risk is dynamically changing. New risk factors emerge (e.g., AIDS), and we must learn to cope with them. Not only does our scientific understanding of specific risks change, but so does the public's values, priorities, and awareness of risks.

Risk may be viewed and evaluated on a worldwide basis over periods of time. If one does this, one sees the climates out of which society's anxieties grow as well as how perceptions change. As a consequence of the increased awareness of drug safety within Western society, an increasing number of drugs have been removed from the market in the past decade.

Reasons given for drug withdrawal from the market have centered on:

1. Lack of efficacy
2. Poor quality
3. Inappropriate or incorrect information and/or promotion
4. Poor cost-effectiveness ratio
5. Safety problems

Screening of the professional press with help of a computer model and data bank during the past 15 months has shown that safety issues are, by far, the most frequent concern reported.

A prescription for what needs to be done concerning risk analysis includes:

1. Improving adverse drug reaction reporting
2. Standardizing prevalence and incidence calculations
3. Assuring good probability assessments
4. Strengthening pharmacoepidemiology knowledge within the industry

In addition, drug risk appraisal should include evaluation of therapeutic risks on a comparative basis, including judging the severity of the risk of intervention in relation to the outcome of the untreated disease.

As regards the management of both real risk and perceived risk, effective communication was described as a key to handling risk. There must be a move away from addressing simply the medical, scientific, and regulatory communities to addressing also the patients, the public at large, politicians, media, and special interest groups. The language must not be only in medical and scientific terms but must also be patient oriented and commonly understandable. The change to addressing a new public with new language should be accompanied by a new behavior which is proactive, and which embraces dialogue.

The day's presentations concluded with the showing of a 20-minute video describing Ciba-Geigy's year-old program, "Risk Assessment of Drugs – Analysis and Response," commonly called RAD-AR.

The discussion of the day's presentations concentrated on the RAD-AR program. A member of the audience pointed out that the emphasis of RAD-AR is on postmarketing surveillance – and he asked whether the technology of the RAD-AR program was also being applied to premarketing activities such as clinical trials. A Ciba-Geigy leader explained that the concept behind the RAD-AR program should not apply only to postmarketing activities but should also apply to clinical and other very early trials. He stressed that RAD-AR concepts encompass both the drugs already on the market as well as those in the premarketing stage.

One speaker suggested that the RAD-AR program should involve regulatory authorities. The company responded by saying that although, of course, collaboration with others in the field is absolutely necessary, first the pharmaceutical companies must meet to exchange ideas – hence, the need for this conference.

Another participant pointed out that there may be excessive focus on quantification of risk, compared to the often neglected quantification of benefit. He asked how the RAD-AR program was attempting to deliver the correct message with regard to the benefits. The answer was that 1 year ago members of Ciba-Geigy met with 20 leading scientists who are knowledgeable in the field of quantifying benefits – in social, quality-of-life, and cost-effectiveness terms. A book entitled *Socioeconomic Evaluation of Drug Therapy* has since been published as a result of that conference.[1] Company leaders feel, however, that evaluating and quantifying benefits of drugs should be performed by each company for its own products, although there are appropriate areas for collaboration.

It was pointed out that while RAD-AR fills an important gap in the evaluation of drugs, it should be aimed at the *average* use of drugs in the real world and not an ideal situation such as is examined in clinical trials. This observation prompted a question from the audience regarding what – if not the real world – the company had been aiming at. The response from the company was that it is possible to become too immersed in medical, scientific, and pharmacological analysis and too far removed from common sense. RAD-AR was aimed at opening windows to the "real world" outside management and the company and making risk assessment of drugs more accurate.

On a more philosophical note, one participant wondered why withdrawals had started to accelerate during the past 5 years. Was it mainly because of a less friendly attitude toward innovation, or was it because there is less tolerance of side effects? Should it be viewed as mainly a negative or a positive phenomenon?

A pharmaceutical representative with regulatory experience described what he called "a variety of reasons" for the acceleration. Sensitivity to environment and medical issues had increased. Additionally, since the early 1960s the pharmaceutical industry and research-based industry have lost leadership to the leading universities. Industry has not been able to keep pace with the evolution of modern drug evaluation technology. Also, during the mid 1970s, pharmaceutical industry leaders often appeared defensive when people from academe, industry, regulatory agencies, and even public interest groups came together to discuss drug problems. There has been a shift in opinion leadership away from the pharmaceutical industry, a shift which will be difficult to reverse, he said.

---

[1] Springer-Verlag Berlin Heidelberg 1988

Part II

Benefit/Risk Analysis and Appraisal

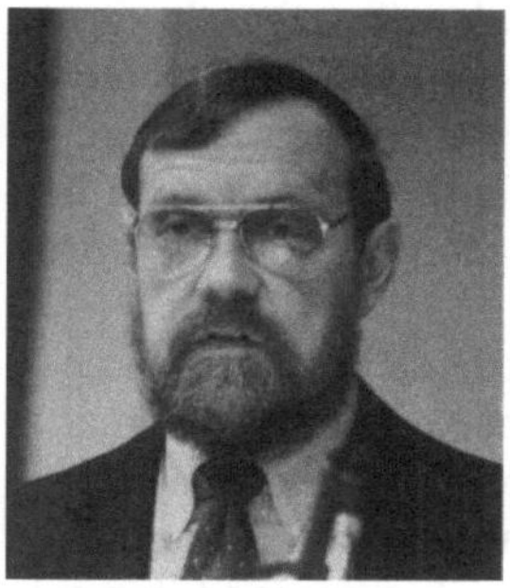

6. Limitations of Available Sources of Data on Prescription Drug Safety

H. A. GUESS

At the time of initial marketing approval, most drugs will have been studied in a few thousand patients treated under carefully controlled protocols designed to evaluate efficacy for specific indications. Such trials generally provide an adequate characterization of the more common types of adverse experiences that may be expected in a population of 1000–5000 patients treated for several months. Adverse effects occurring only with long-term use cannot usually be quantitated since typically only a few hundred patients will have been treated for a year or more. Ethical constraints also limit the extent to which clinical trial treatment experience can be accumulated in special populations such as pregnant women, the very elderly, neonates, and patients with impaired renal, hepatic, or cardiovascular function. Because of these limitations, very rare adverse reactions or drug interactions, adverse effects occurring mainly in certain high-risk populations, teratogenic effects, and adverse effects becoming evident only after long-term use cannot usually be examined [1].

To some extent a knowledge of the clinical pharmacology of a new compound may help identify adverse effects related to the basic mechanism of action of the drug. However, for idiosyncratic effects, structure does not always predict patterns of toxicity. For example, the molecular structures of brompheniramine and zimelidine are quite similar and their empirical formulas are nearly identical (B. E. Wilholm, personal communication), yet their patterns of toxicity differ in a way that did not become fully apparent until zimelidine was marketed [9]. Brompheniramine maleate is a widely used nontoxic antihistamine. Zimelidine is an antidepressant that was withdrawn from the market in Sweden because it greatly increased the risk of Guillain-Barré syndrome (GBS) [9].

The incidence of GBS among recipients of zimeldine was estimated to be about 23-fold higher than the incidence in the general population of Sweden (about 2.5 cases per 100000 persons per year) [9]. Although one case of GBS was reported in a zimeldine recipient during clinical trials, the relationship of this disorder to zimeldine was not fully recognized until additional cases were reported with marketed use of the drug. The failure to appreciate the relationship between zimeldine and GBS on the basis of a single case reported in clinical trials is understandable since GBS is typically idiopathic, not often imputed to drug therapy, and is only one of many rare disorders of uncertain etiology occurring sporadically in the general population.

This example illustrates some of the difficulties to be faced in assessing the significance of one or two isolated cases of a rare disorder encountered in clinical trials of a new drug. The limited number of patients treated in clinical trials means that the most likely outcome for many rare adverse effects is for no cases to occur, and the next most likely outcome is for one or two isolated cases to occur under circumstances where a causal relationship to the study drug may seem rather unlikely. Thus, it is to be expected that most rare adverse drug effects will first become apparent after marketing.

The sources of information on drug safety after marketing can be broadly grouped into four categories: voluntary spontaneous adverse experience reports to the manufacturer or regulatory agencies; case reports in the medical literature; postmarketing surveillance studies including both company-sponsored phase IV studies and the prescription-event monitoring (PEM) studies pioneered by Inman; and formal epidemiologic case-control studies. While case reports in the medical literature have played a valuable role in primary alerting to rare new adverse drug reactions [10], the lack of reliable numerator and denominator information makes it impossible to quantify risks or, in many cases, to separate chance associations from events that are causally related to the drug in question.

Spontaneous adverse experience reports likewise provide a valuable mechanism for alerting one to rare but serious adverse drug reactions. Indeed, for highly unusual illnesses spontaneous reporting is presently the only way in which the potential relationship to drug therapy can be studied in a timely manner. On the other hand, the limitations of spontaneous adverse experience reporting have been well documented [2]. Not only is the case reporting incomplete, but the extent of under-reporting is so unpredictable as to make any safety comparisons between drugs on the basis of spontaneous reporting of questionable validity. In two of the few instances in which the extent of under-reporting could be verified against essentially complete ascertainment of cases, a reporting rate of 35% (29/84) was found for hospitalized cases of drug-associated neutropenia in Sweden [3] and 12.5% (4/32) for fatal blood dyscrasias associated with phenylbutazone in the United Kingdom [4]. When the overall rate of spontaneous reporting of angioedema with the angiotensin converting enzyme inhibitor enalapril was compared to that seen in three large postmarketing studies in which relatively complete case ascertainment could be expected, the approximate spontaneous reporting rate (1 case in 10000 patients treated) was about one-tenth that in the studies (1 case in 1000 patients treated) [5].

Weber [6] showed that for nonsteroidal anti-inflammatory drugs studied in the United Kingdom during the late 1970s, the rate of reporting was higher in the first few years of marketing than in subsequent years. During the early 1980s, however, there was a steady upward trend in adverse drug experience reporting to the United States Food and Drug Administration (FDA)), even with older drugs [2]. Thus, as Rossi et al. [2] noted, any attempt to apply Weber's findings to drugs initially marketed in the United States during the early 1980s would have to incorporate an additional correction for the upward trend of overall increased reporting during this time period. If one were to consider the additional fact that any adjustment factor must itself have inherent variability (which may be impossible to quantitate), it should be clear that no statistical manipulations can fully compensate for the many vagaries of spontaneous reporting. Comparisons between drugs on the basis of such data are highly suspect, at best. A few of the many additional factors that have been mentioned as having an important effect on completeness of spontaneous reporting include the severity, timing, and uniqueness of the reaction; whether the reaction is mentioned in the manufacturer's prescribing information; publicity surrounding the adverse reaction; the way in which the manufacturer's sales representatives deal with adverse reactions in their discussions with physicians; and physician interest in reporting.

In addition to problems with completeness of case reporting, there is also the problem of adequacy of the medical information in the reports themselves. All too often the initial reports are too incomplete to be medically useful, and follow-up information may be impossible to obtain. All of these limitations lead to the conclusion that spontaneous adverse experience reports and case reports in the medical literature are good for raising questions about drug safety but are poor sources of data for answering them.

Postmarketing surveillance studies are an additional source of safety information for newly marketed drugs. In the typical phase IV studies, between 5000 and 20000 patients are treated with the drug in ordinary clinical practice and are followed for a period of time to document the time on therapy and the occurrence of adverse experiences while on therapy [7]. By extending the base of clinical trial experience with a new drug such studies can provide additional assurance of safety for possibly drug-related disorders that have an expected rate of occurrence of about 0.1%. Such disorders could be missed in clinical trials or, more likely, would appear as a few isolated cases with uncertain causality. In a population of 10000 patients treated, it is likely that either one would see enough cases to permit a useful clinical and statistical assessment of risk, or one would see no further cases, thereby increasing the confidence that the original cases were not drug related. This view defines what a phase IV study might be expected to do under the best of circumstances,

In practice, however, things are not so clear-cut. When one follows any population of several thousand patients for several months, a number of untoward medical events can be expected to occur. In the absence of a carefully chosen control group, it is not possible to determine which events are causally related to the drug under study and which are not. Even with a control group this task may still be impossible because of the difficulty of achieving adequate comparability between the patients on treatment and the control group. Lawson [8] has described these problems clearly, based on his own experience with a large post marketing surveillance study of cimetidine.

PEM offers an alternative to the usual phase IV studies. The typical sample size of a PEM study is about the same as that of a phase IV study. In the PEM studies, events are monitored while the patients are on the study drug and after discontinuation of the study drug. By comparing the rates of events on therapy with the rates of events after discontinuation of therapy, there is the expectation that hypotheses can be generated about unknown adverse drug reactions. These studies have proven useful in the study of several newly marketed drugs. However, it is still very difficult to sort out truly drug-related events from events that would be expected to occur in the patient population under study apart from any association with the drug being monitored.

Case-control studies have been used to quantitate rare or delayed effects (both harmful and protective) of widely used drugs such as oral contraceptives. The Slone Epidemiology Unit of Boston University has published a number of such studies. On the other hand, case-control studies are presently not well suited to the study of rare effects of newly marketed drugs. The reason is a matter of arithmetic, best illustrated by example. Suppose that in its 1st year of marketing drug X is suspected of causing rare horrid syndrome Y in patients aged 65 years and older. Let us assume that the "background rate" of horrid syndrome Y in the general United States population aged 65 and older is one case per 15000 persons per year. Further assume that during its first year of marketing, 0.8% of the United States population aged 65 and older has been treated with the drug. Using these data one can calculate that a minimum of 113 cases of horrid syndrome Y would have to be assembled for a case-control study with sufficient statistical power to detect a fivefold elevation of risk in horrid syndrome Y among users of drug X aged 65 and older relative to the risk in the general population of people of the same age. (Here we are using a one-tailed test with $\alpha = 0.05$, $\beta = 0.20$, and assuming ten controls per case.) To assemble such cases, one would have to have access to medical diagnoses on about 1.7 million persons (113×15000) aged 65 and older. Without some form of computer-based medical records linkage system, the task of locating enough cases would be insurmountable if the study results were needed within several months.

Although the above example is hypothetical, the parameters are close to an actual case of a drug that was withdrawn from the market. Definitive investigation of the suspected rare side effect was impossible to conduct in time to meet regulatory demands for action. This example illustrates a general fact about investigating rare side effects of newly marketed drugs using case control studies. The number of cases one must assemble to make a finding of "no increased risk" statistically convincing is often so large as to make the study infeasible. At first glance it might seem that this problem could be avoided by conducting a cohort study of users of the drug rather than a case-control study. However, for very rare events, cohort studies would often need to be so large as also to be infeasible without use of a computer-based records linkage system. In the above example, a cohort study of about 30000 patients aged 65 and older treated with drug X and a control group of the same size, both followed for 1 year, would be needed to provide the same power of detecting a fivefold risk increase as the above case-control study.

Over the past two decades a number of computer-based medical records linkage systems have come into being in the United States and Canada as parts of administrative and financial record-keeping systems for either prepaid medical plans or health insurance plans. Typically these systems provide a computer record of at least all prescriptions and all hospital discharge diagnoses for all members of the covered population over some extended time period. Through use of unique patient identification numbers, the prescription and hospitalization records can be linked on a patient-by-patient basis to create for each patient a complete chronological record of each prescription filled and each hospitalization. While not designed as data sources for epidemiologic studies, these systems have been widely hailed as having the potential for providing rapid access to the information needed to study safety questions with newly marketed drugs. With few exceptions, however, the potential has not been realized. Operational difficulties have been many and have included data quality, cost, limited population size, limited formulary coverage, difficulties in obtaining abstracted data from the original medical records to supplement the diagnostic codes available on the computer file, confidentiality concerns, and the ability to assemble and support qualified research staffs with interest in conducting epidemiologic studies with such data.

Perhaps the most productive medical records linkage system incorporating both pharmacy and hospital records has been that maintained by the Puget Sound Group Health Cooperative, a health maintenance organization (HMO) with about 320000 subscribers. This records linkage system has been used extensively by the Boston Collaborative Drug Surveillance Program headed by Jick and Walker [11]. However, the limited formulary of this HMO and the relatively small population size limit the ability of this system to provide useful data on suspected rare adverse effects of newly marketed drugs.

In the United States each state administers a social insurance program, known as Medicaid, for the poor. These separately administered programs provide payment to physicians and hospitals who treat patients eligible for coverage. Billing records for prescription drugs and medical services are maintained on computer files and can be linked within each state by patient identification numbers. Several different groups have developed medical linkage systems based on Medicaid data. The largest is the COMPASS system operated by a private company (Health Information Designs) with major funding support from a contract with the FDA. Approximately seven million patients are covered in this system. Several epidemiologic studies of adverse drug effects have been published by Strom and Carson using this data base [12]. One of the problems with the COMPASS system is that copies of medical records have been difficult to retrieve in a timely manner. Several other problems with Medicaid data have been outlined by Faich [13].

Medicaid information for Tennessee includes about 400000 eligible patients and has been used for epidemiologic studies by Ray and others in the Department of Preventive Medicine at Vanderbilt University [14]. While copies of medical records are readily available for this population, the small size limits the ability to study very rare adverse effects of newly marketed drugs.

Between 1975 and 1987, the province of Saskatchewan in Canada maintained computer records of all prescriptions, all hospitalizations, all cancer diagnoses, and all deaths for nearly all residents of the province. Over 95% of the one million residents were covered by this plan. Those excluded were covered by federal plans and included native North Americans, federal personnel, and inmates of correctional institutes. The records were linkable by unique patient identification numbers. Copies of the medical records were readily available for review. One epidemiologic study using this data base was recently published [15], and several others by other university and industry groups are in progress. In July 1987 the province changed from a reimbursement program, in which all prescriptions were reimbursed, to one in which reimbursement was provided only when a familiy-specific, deductible amount had been exceeded. In conjunction with this the provincial authorities decided to index prescriptions only to the level of the family, not to the level of the individual. This meant that only six of the eight digits of the patient identifier had to be entered into the computer. Also the prescriptions were entered only after the familiy-specific deductible amount had been met. These changes have probably resulted in some cost savings for data entry. However, they eliminated the ability to study adverse effects of prescription drugs in Saskatchewan.

Prior to its effective dismantlement, this was the largest medical records linkage system in North America (and possibly in the world) covering an entire geographic area with a population of one million persons and providing for timely retrieval of original medical records. The example of what was done in Saskatchewan illustrates the political and administrative difficulties in maintaining and operating medical records linkage systems that can be used for epidemiologic studies.

Any viable plan for the management and perception of prescription drug risks must address the as yet unsolved problem of measuring risks of suspected rare but serious adverse effects of newly marketed drugs in a timely manner. It is difficult to manage risks when one cannot place useful upper bounds on how large the risks are likely to be. Because of the sample size requirements, computer-based medical records linkage systems offer perhaps the only practical method for doing this. The task of communicating a better understanding of risks and benefits of prescription drugs might well begin with an effort to increase the understanding within the medical community of the value of maintaining sources of epidemiologic data necessary to study risks and benefits of newly marketed drugs in a timely manner. To date, the pharmaceutical industry has provided limited funds for ongoing research by individual groups working with such systems. Emergency funding for "crash" studies has also been provided on occasion. However, there has not been a sustained, unified industry commitment for establishment and operation of medical records linkage systems of sufficient size and quality to be useful for measuring risks of suspected rare adverse effects of newly marketed drugs. Such a commitment is needed. More timely data would benefit the entire medical community, most of all the patients.

References

1. Faich GA (1986) Adverse drug reaction monitoring. N Engl J Med 314: 1589–1592
2. Rossi AC, Hsu JP, Faich GA (1987) Ulcerogenicity of piroxicam: an analysis of spontaneously reported data. Br Med J 294: 147–150
3. Arneborn P, Palmblad J (1982) Drug-induced neutropenia – A survey for Stockholm: 1973–1978. Acta Med Scand 212: 289–292
4. Inman WHW (1977) Study of fatal bone marrow depression with special reference to phenylbutazone and oxyphenbutazone. Br Med J 1500–1505
5. Slater EE et al. (1988) Clinical profile or angioedema associated with angiotensin converting enzyme inhibition. JAMA 260: 967–970
6. Weber JCP (1984) Epidemiology of adverse reactions to nonsteroidal anti-inflammatory drugs. In: Rainsford KD, Velo GP (eds) Advances in inflammation research. Raven, New York
7. Hagler L, et al. (1987) A primer of post-marketing surveillance. Drug Inform J 21: 69–107
8. Lawson DH (1987) Post-marketing surveillance: the problems in practice. In: Mann RD (ed) Adverse drug reactions. Parthenon, Park Ridge NJ, pp 159–164
9. Fagius A, Ostermann PO, Sidén A, Wilholm BE (1985) Guillain-Barré syndrome following zimeldine treatment. J Neurol Neurosurg Psychiatry 48: 65–69
10. Venning GR (1983) Identification of adverse reactions to new drugs (parts I–IV). Br Med J 286: 199–202, 289–292, 365–368, 458–460, 544–547
11. Jick H (1985) Use of automated data bases to study drug effects after marketing. Pharmacotherapy 5: 278–279
12. Strom BL, Carson JL, Morse ML, LeRoy A (1985) The computerized on-line Medicaid pharmaceutical analysis and surveillance system (COMPASS) – a new resource for post-marketing surveillance. Clin Pharmacol Ther 38: 359–364
13. Faich GA (1986) Post-marketing surveillance of prescription drugs: current status. Clinical Medicine Research Institute, New York
14. Ray WA, Griffin MR, Schaffner W, Baugh DK, Melton LJ III (1987) Psychotropic drug use and the risk of hip fracture. N Engl J Med 316: 363–369
15. Guess HA, West R, Strand LM, Helston D, Lydick EG, Bergman U, Wolski K (1988) Fatal upper gastrointestinal hemorrhage or perforation among users and nonusers of nonsteroidal anti-inflammatory drugs in Saskatchewan, Canada 1983. J Clin Epidemiol 41: 35–45

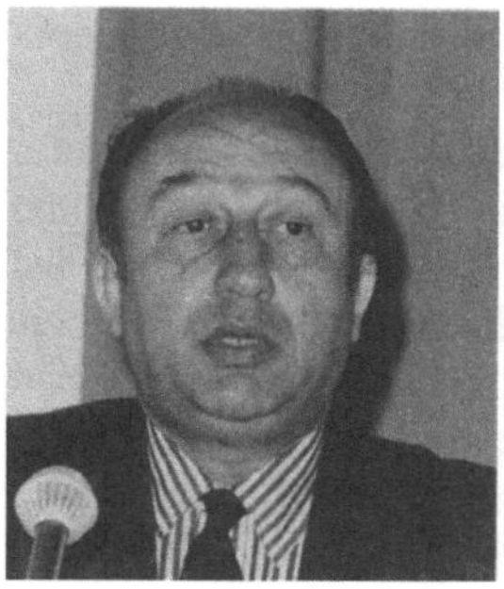

7. Strategies, Designs, Criteria, Tactics and Statistics to be Considered when Evaluating Scientific Evidence

Introduction: What Is Epidemiology?

Most accepted definitions of epidemiology in standard textbooks and as taught by leading professors throughout North America are consistent with the following: Epidemiology is the study of the determinants of health and disease in human populations; it subsumes the study of distribution of health-related phenomena in man.

Historically, epidemiology started with the study of epidemics of infections or communicable diseases such as cholera, smallpox and influenza. An epidemic is defined simply as an unusually high frequency of a disease. An epidemic can last days or weeks, which is common for most communicable disease epidemics, or it can last decades, as in tuberculosis or, more characteristically, in non-communicable or chronic diseases. For instance, we have been in the upward curve regarding the incidence of lung cancer for decades. Happily for mankind, it appears that the epidemic of cardiovascular diseases, also lasting for decades, has peaked, and we are now on the downward side of the curve. During the past 12–15 years the mortality attributable to cardiovascular disease has diminished by approximately 25% in most Western countries. Curiously, no one, not even the best experts, is sure why mortality due to cardiovascular diseases is declining, although many hypotheses have been advanced.

The quintessence of the challenge for the epidemiologist is the elucidation of causes of disease, or, conversely, of factors explaining the preservation of health. In our context, adverse drug reactions can be equated with disease. Epidemiologic principles are directly applicable to evaluation of possible adverse drug reactions. It was an epidemiologist who first found convincing evidence in humans linking cigarette smoking with cancer of the lung in a cause-and-effect relationship. Epidemiologic principles have addressed such controversies in the pharmacological sciences as the risk of oral contraceptives, the relationship between thalidomide and congenital deformities, and the association between breast cancer and reserpine.

There are certain rules of the game or certain criteria that must be met in order to establish a cause-and-effect relationship between a risk factor and an alleged disease or adverse reaction. Showing a statistical relationship or a statistical association between a risk factor and a disease is not sufficient; there are further requirements that must be satisfied before deciding that a statistical association indeed represents causation.

Epidemiology is one of the branches of biomedical science. There are certain criteria for the admissibility of the science done under the aegis of epidemiology which are unique to the field; such work is seldom done in the same way in other branches of the health sciences. For instance, workers in other fields seldom engage in projects called case-control studies; the methods used for case-control studies are prescribed almost exclusively by epidemiologists. However, most of the methodological considerations in scientific work of epidemiology are common to research in other health sciences and for science in general. For instance, the need for control groups in studies trying to establish cause or seeking to show the effectiveness of an intervention is not uniquely epidemiologic; it is a basic requirement of any biomedical science.

In order for the results of research to be declared valid, several fundamental criteria for the conduct of research must be observed as one produces evidence about a particular research question or hypothesis. In law there are rules of admissibility of evidence; in the health sciences there also are rules of admissibility of evidence. Such rules apply particularly to epidemiologic research concerning pharmaceuticals.

Association Is Not Necessarily Causation

An association between two entities is assessed statistically when an event occurs following exposure to a risk factor more often than in circumstances when the risk factor is not present. If the event following the risk factor happens at such a rate that the excess between occurrence with exposure compared to occurrence without exposure to a risk factor is greater than one might expect by chance alone, there is said to be a statistically significant association. For instance, fatal automobile accidents occur twice as frequently among people who do not wear seat belts as among people who do wear seat belts while driving. This is a stastistical relationship, and it is unlikely to arise by chance when one considers statistics from a whole province or state. However, one cannot automatically assume that not using seat belts is a cause of fatalities through automobile accidents. First, many fatalities occur among people who do, in fact, wear seat belts. Second, not wearing seat belts may simply be one indicator of a driving personality or attitude that makes the driver more prone to accidents. Conceivably, those who do not wear seat belts are also more likely to drink excessively prior to driving. The foregoing example is put forward to show how important it is to discriminate between an observed statistical association between two health-related phenomena and a possible cause-and-effect significance of the same association. What, then, are the considerations when trying to impute causality to an association?

Scientists must constantly remind themselves that association does not mean causation. The most convincing evidence for causation can be obtained only through experimental approaches. Of experimental approaches, the strongest, most reliable evidence for causality is the randomized controlled trial. When experimental evidence is not available, or this approach is not feasible, we must rely on non-experimental evidence.

Experimental Evidence

If the evidence obtained about an association is derived from a true experiment, that is, one in which the investigator has had unbiased discretion over the assignment of study subjects to an experimental arm, on the one hand, and to a control or reference arm on the other, the findings tend to be conclusive. Most evidence in epidemiologic research, however, is not experimental.

Non-Experimental Evidence

Sir Austin Bradford Hill has suggested nine features to consider in looking at associations between factors and outcomes when the evidence is derived from non-experimental methods. These are the following:

Strength. If the exposed population shows the outcome variable in a very marked degree, we are much more comfortable in inferring causation. High odds ratios mean a strong association. Fishermen in the Canadian Province of Newfoundland have a risk ratio or odds ratio of 1.65 in respect to cancer of the lip when the reference group is composed of male Newfoundlanders who are not fishermen. Thus, commercial fishermen in Newfoundland have a 65% higher chance of developing cancer of the lip than non-fisherman. A risk ratio of 1.65 (or, an excess of 65%) is a *weak* association. In contrast, the risk of certain cerebral vascular sequelae among women taking oral contraceptives, compared to women who do not take oral contraceptives, has been reported to be as high as 6 in certain studies. This is a *strong* association. The evidence linking cigarette smoking with cancer of the lung in studies from various countries have ranged from 8 to 23 when measured as odds ratios or risk ratios. These are *very strong* associations. In general, the stronger the association, the more likely that it is causal. But strength alone is not sufficient to reach a verdict of causality. Of course, sometimes we are misled. A very strong association between two factors may be *merely* a strong association and not an instance of cause and effect at all. For oral contraceptives, it now appears that risk is most strongly related to the progestin component of earlier formulations, and risk associated with current formulations is much lower (and poorly studied).

Consistency. If the statistical relationship between two health-related entities has been shown, has this been the case in more than one study? With different designs? Was it demonstrated in the hands of more than one investigator? In more than one place? Under different circumstances and at different times? Risk ratios or odds ratios summarizing statistical relationships that are found consistently in different parts of the world with different investigators using a similar technique but in different circumstances tend to support the notion that the relationship is causal. The criteria of consistency places great weight on similar results reached from quite different designs. It is more convincing than similar results from a collection of similarly designed studies. Weakly designed studies all pointing in the same direction have frequently misled us into believing causation when, in fact, the same mistake was simply being repeated. This may have been the pattern in the reserpine and breast cancer controversy. On the other hand, the connection between smoking and lung cancer has been observed repeatedly by different workers in different countries using quite different populations over many years. The case for causality in these observed associations became increasingly strong with each new study.

Specificity. If the association is unusual, if it is limited to specifically exposed persons who develop unusual outcomes, there is a strong argument in favour of causation. In other words, if the statistical association is limited to specifically delineated study subjects in particular settings, and if the association is confined to certain types of diseases or health phenomena, and if, on the other hand, one does not show an association between people in these similar settings and other target health phenomena or diseases, then there is an argument in favour of causation. The peculiar form of deformity produced by exposure of pregnant women to thalidomide and the association between acquired immune-deficiency syndrome and the generally very rare Kaposi's sarcoma are recent examples of evidential specificity for causation. However, lack of specificity is an argument that should be invoked against causality with extreme caution. There can be many different possible causes for a particular disease; there are also many single factors which can cause more than one disease.

Temporality. From common sense we know it to be highly implausible that an effect precedes its cause. But confusion in this regard cannot automatically be prevented even among investigators. Does a particular occupation or occupational environment promote infection by the tubercle bacillus, or are the people who select this kind of work more liable to contract tuberculosis, whatever the environment – or, indeed, have they already contracted it? When certain epidemiologic studies are done, the key issue to remember is that the way in which the data have been gathered and the format in which they are presented do not always allow a confident decision on the sequence of two health-related facts which one is trying to relate. In the question of whether sour gas emissions from the natural gas industry of Alberta were a potential cause of respiratory conditions, one must ask whether people had upper respiratory symptoms before or after exposure to those emissions. They may only remember the health effects following the time they were exposed, and it is a real challenge to determine whether there were any changes in the intensity and the frequency of these health perceptions before and after exposure.

Biologic Gradients/Dose-Response Relationships. If the association or the relationship is one in which one can show a biological gradient or a dose-response curve, the argument for causation is strengthened. For example, if adverse health effects from radiation are greatest near the epicentre of a radiation source and diminish progressively as the exposed persons become more distant from the radiation source, such findings militate for a causal interpretation of any relationships or associations observed. Those who smoke more cigarettes have a higher death rate from smoking than both non-smokers and those who smoke but a few cigarettes.

Reverse Gradient/Reversibility. Evidence of a reverse gradient, that is, if the frequency of the intensity of the adverse health effect is reduced upon discontinuance of exposure, can be regarded as having as much strength as that of a positive gradient.

For example, rates of lung cancer and cardiovascular disease among smokers fall after cessation of smoking.

Biologic Plausibility. Sometimes it can be shown that certain events are related to one another only with statistical significance. If the association seems to make no sense at all, as in a relationship between the number of Presbyterian ministers in Scotland and the increasing population in Chicago or the number of bathrooms in women's homes, we should be cautious in inferring causation. Even the most uninitiated lay person will immediately recognize how biologically or clinically implausible it is to think of bathrooms causing breast cancer. However, it is a known phenomenon that women with higher socio-economic status have more cancer of the breast. Women with higher socio-economic status also tend to have more bathrooms in their homes than women of lower socio-economic status. Thus, the double relationship of socio-economic status with both breast cancer and number of bathrooms suggests an association which is obviously *spurious* even if statistically significant. In evaluating observed associations, whether statistically significant or not, the biological and clinical plausibility must always be taken into account. However, overemphasis on this consideration must be avoided because, as science advances, what is not biologically plausible today may become plausible tomorrow in the light of new knowledge. When Prof. Oliver Wendell Holmes of the Harvard Medical School in 1847 drew attention to the association between the hand-washing habits of obstetrical surgeons and the incidence of puerperal fever, no one paid much attention because they could see no biological plausibility in the association. Twenty years later, after the work of Pasteur and Lister, the association became clearly plausible.

Coherence of the Evidence. Reaching a conclusion of causality for a particular association should not be at variance with generally known and accepted theories in biology and general science. There should be coherence about what is otherwise known of the natural history, relationships, the biology and the physical sciences undergirding the phenomena under consideration. This must be considered cautiously at any stage of scientific evolution. John Snow's historical epidemiologic observations on the transmission of cholera by the water from the Broad Street pump in London were controversial and at variance with many prevailing therories of the time; yet they would have been beyond question had the organism concerned already been isolated (which did not happen until three or four decades later). The association of lung cancer and cigarette smoking is coherent with the increase in smoking among men that occurred between 1910 and 1920 and the later increase among women. The isolation of carcinogenic factors from cigarette smoke and the histopathologic evidence of irritation of the airway epithelium of heavy smokers lend further evidence of coherence.

Analogy. As a subordinate but nevertheless important consideration, in some circumstances it is appropriate to use analogy when reasoning through the clinical significance of observed associations. For instance, if a particular drug had caused a particular type of genetic malformation, and a second drug of similar molecular composition is suspected to have similar teratogenic effects, such an analogy accompanied by other criteria presented earlier in this section would militate for causation.

However, *the absence of analogy does not rule out causality, and the presence of it does not rule it in.* For example, since sigmoidoscopic examinations prevent cancer of the colon and rectum by enabling removal of suspicious polyps, the examination of stools for occult blood ought to have the same preventive effect and cause a similar reduction of death from cancer of the colon. However, this reduction has not been proven. Analogy is to be invoked with extreme caution in causal reasoning or in inference about causality from observed associations.

In summary, for causation we prefer to have evidence from a soundly conceived and executed experiment – one that employs the appropriate strengthening factors of random allocation to treatment and employs appropriate varieties of blindness on the part of the experimenter, the patient, the evaluator of the outcome, and even the statistician who analyses the data. When experimental evidence is not available or is feasible to obtain, we must rely on non-experimental evidence to assess relationships for cause and effect. None of the nine criteria used for non-experimental evidence is sufficient by itself to arrive at a verdict of causation from association. One generally requires that a majority of the nine criteria point in the direction of causation before risking a verdict of causation. It should be clear that in the presence of a statistical association, an arbitrary decision on biostatistical significance is not sufficient for drawing causal conclusions. Moreover, overdependence on statistical significance can be misleading or frankly erroneous.

Lastly, the information utilized to make inferences and reason through the causal significance of observed associations must depend on well-designed, well-executed and soundly analysed studies. Criteria of admissibility of evidence must be respected. One cannot reach good decisions about cause-and-effect relationships from research studies of substandard quality, particularly if the data are known to be invalid for whatever reason.

Rules of Scientific Admissibility of Evidence

A scientific study which seeks to establish cause-and-effect types of relationships or to evaluate the effectiveness of an intervention must follow certain general rules to be able to provide scientifically admissible evidence.

Research Questions, Hypotheses, and Statistical Analyses Should Be Specified in Advance

Unless a study is only exploratory, or unless a study involves post hoc secondary analyses to generate hypotheses for subsequent projects, the research questions and hypotheses of a particular study must be set forth clearly and *in advance* of any field work or analysis. Such research questions must be formulated in a manner that permits quantitative answers.

It is irresponsible for an investigator to embark on a study, even if it involves only analysis of existing data, without preparing a protocol, or a written, documented research plan. Such a plan should be evaluated by peer scientists before it is implemented, particularly if it requires funds from public sources. An ethics review should generally be part of the evaluation process and is absolutely essential if the study involves human subjects in any way. Once the study gets underway, deviations from the study plan or protocol should be documented and justified.

One should not depend on statistical analysis to correct for lack of quality of data at source. In particular, no conceivable statistical analysis using correlations, regression, etc., can offset the lack of control groups or reference groups. A lack of control group or reference group renders a study inadmissible in the study of cause-and-effect relationship or of effectiveness (unless the analysis is on dose-response within a cohort, in which case a part of the cohort is effectively serving as the "control").

Methodological Requirements

All of the following methodological issues should be considered in planning the study rather than after study completion, with statistical adjustment of the data. The eligibility and ineligibility of study subjects to be assessed must be clearly specified. The method of sampling must be clearly specified and justified. Sample sizes must be justified, and statistical power should be demonstrated. Experimental and control groups (or reference groups) must be carefully chosen and must be representative of the totality of the subjects under consideration. The investigators must give objective criteria of evaluation of the dependent or target variables with extensive description of the measurement techniques employed. The independent variables must also be carefully delineated. Observer variation and selection bias must be taken into account. Possible confounding variables must be considered and accounted for. Attrition of subjects must be anticipated and sample size calculations adjusted accordingly. Response rates must be high, and rates below 90% for most population studies must be carefully justified.

The foregoing are important but not exhaustive considerations. A general principle is that *reproducible* criteria for choice of subjects, for measurement of phenomena of importance, for classification of interventions, etc., must be declared in advance of the execution of a project.

Reproducibility and Verifiability

For a study or a scientific project to be admissible it should be possible for comparably qualified investigators either to replicate the study in other settings and obtain similar results or, at the very least, to verify the analyses and calculations from the same basic data employed by the original investigators. Unless a study is replicable and verifiable, it should be considered inadmissible.

Naturally, the exact structure of a protocol and the precise details of the plan depend on the type of study being proposed. This is different for an experimental study and for non-experimental designs such as cohort studies, case-control studies, surveys, cross-sectional studies and uncontrolled case series. However, in imputing causality to an exposure factor with respect to a health outcome, it is important to establish the hierarchy of strength of evidence from the different kinds of studies; in descending order these are:

1. Experimental studies, such as randomized controlled trials.
2. Cohort analytic studies, that is, studies with two or more cohorts being compared concurrently or historically.
3. Case-control studies (also called case-referent studies), which for very rare diseases provide evidence of good quality and are therefore applicable to the study of rare adverse drug reactions.
4. Cross-sectional studies may be important to deal with the question, "Is there a problem?" but, by definition, such studies cannot establish or rule out causation.
5. All uncontrolled studies are hypothesis-generating or descriptive studies, unless one is dealing with highly dramatic findings. For instance, controlled studies were not necessary to evaluate the effectiveness of penicillin when it was discovered; conditions that had been normally fatal were cured overnight.

All these types of studies are used in pharmaceutical research. Phase I studies usually employ uncontrolled cohort studies. It is now usually expected that phase II and III studies be controlled clinical trials. Cohort and case-control studies are generally used in phase IV to address post-marketing issues, including evaluation of adverse drug reactions.

Experimental Design

An experimental design is one in which one group of eligible subjects or patients exposed to an intervention or a manoeuvre is compared to one or more control groups comparable to the intervention groups in all respects, save for the intervention or manoeuvre of interest. The essential characteristic of an experiment is that the intervention or the manoeuvre is assigned by the investigator to the exposed group, and that the comparison interventions or manoeuvres (e.g. placebo or the best accepted current therapy) are also assigned by the investigator to the control group or control groups. Thus the assignment of manoeuvres is under unbiased control of the investigator.

Generally an investigator in such circumstances chooses to assign subjects randomly to the intervention or the control group. However, it is possible to have controlled studies that do not use random assignment or allocation of subjects to treatment groups, but are still experimental. The assignment may be done in a systematic fashion by other preselected means (e.g. alternate assignment rules or odd versus even hospital file numbers) or, conceivably, on a judgmental basis. In our current understanding of clinical science, the experiment which is a randomized controlled trial is the "gold standard" of research.

I prefer to call designs in which the investigator does not control the assignment of study subjects to treated versus untreated groups by the term non-experimental. There are several equivalent terms which one finds in the literature for non-experimental, designs; these include: subexperimental, quasi-experimental, or observational. The term quasi-experimental is not acceptable because a design either does or does not meet criteria to be deemed experimental. The term observational is also unacceptable because the word incorrectly suggests that experimental designs do not involve observation of phenomena.

Cohort Design

The word *cohort,* from the Latin, is a Roman military term and referred to a group of soldiers of a certain category; for example, 100 or 500 infantrymen, cavalry, etc. Its most important use in clinical and epidemiologic research is to designate a number of persons (patients or healthy individuals) who share common attributes considered relevant to the research questions at issue. For example, this could be 500 persons aged 20–49, experiencing a first episode of low back pain, who have no clinically objective signs of neurological deficit. The cohort might be 10000 diabetics aged 50–79 eligible for inclusion by definite criteria and unaffected by peripheral vascular complications.

Sometimes the only intervention or manoeuvre of interest in studying a cohort is the passage of time, or the natural history of a condition. Thus, for diabetics unaffected by peripheral vascular complications, one might wish to discover how many complications affect this population of diabetics over a 5-year period. One might study a new drug recently introduced into the market to delay or prevent peripheral vascular complications and seek to determine the rate of development of such complications in a cohort of persons using the drug.

For any cohort, it is important to determine in advance the dependent variable or the target outcome. The outcome events become the numerators for rates calculated in cohort studies (such as incidence). For survivors of liver transplants, the dependent variable or target outcome might be death. For a cohort of patients with rheumatoid arthritis given a new drug, it might be length of time to the next flare-up of their disease. The fundamental characteristic of the cohort is that the study subjects are identified and delineated by explicit criteria *before* the declared target outcome or dependent variable of interest is manifest among the same subjects. Cohorts are denominators for target outcomes. The target outcomes or dependent variables are the numerators. *In cohort studies, the denominators are always identified and delineated before the dependent variables are observed.*

Cohorts may be followed in time as a single group without making any comparisons with any other group. Such work is referred to as descriptive or, more specifically, a single-cohort study or an uncontrolled cohort study. Sometimes it is possible to compare two or more cohorts and follow them simultaneously. For instance, it may be possible to assemble 20000 men who became exposed and continue to be exposed to occupationally related radiation in nuclear plants and to follow these men from say, 1971 to 1995 to determine the total number of new cancers. This could be done at the same time as one follows another 20000 men in other energy-related industries, similar in most respects to nuclear power plants except for the exposure to measured levels of radiation in the workplace. Note why this is not an experimental design: the investigator did not assign the men to be or to not be exposed to radiation – the men were self-selected. However, it should be established that the two self-selected cohorts are sufficiently comparable to follow them forward in time and compare the rate of development of new cancers between the two groups. With two or more groups, we have a cohort-analytic study or a cohort-comparison study. It is worth emphasizing that all 40000 men were free of the target outcome of interest (cancer) at the time the cohorts were assembled in 1971.

The main disadvantage of cohort studies is that they generally require very large numbers of subjects in the denominator so that meaningful numbers in the numerator (target outcome) can emerge as dependent variables. The precision of the answers depends greatly on the size of the numerator. A prominent potential source of bias exists in disease or target outcome ascertainment, i. e. determination of occurrences of the outcome of interest. Also, cohort studies sometimes require long follow-up with all the consequent problems of logistics and cost, the most important one being losses to follow-up.

Case-Control Design

The case-control design is a special case of the cross-sectional approach. Cross-sectional designs, in general, are those in which denominators, or groups of subjects, are delineated at the same time that numerator events (target outcomes, disease) are measured. Cross-sectional studies are more vulnerable to bias and misinterpretation than cohort studies, in which measurement of target outcomes is more controlled because it is defined in advance and measured prospectively. However, due to reasons of budget, unavailability of data, unavailability of time or ethical constraints, a cohort study very often cannot be done, and all that one can do is a cross-sectional study. It is important to stress that when data emerge only from cross-sectional studies, one can only reach tentative conclusions that a particular exposure factor or intervention is *associated* with a particular target outcome. Causal conclusions are not warranted.

Tactically, the distinct feature of the case-control study is that the two groups compared, the group of cases and the subjects from the control group, are demarcated by the presence or absence of the target outcome of interest. One then determines, in each of the two groups compared, how frequently an exposure of interest occurred. For instance, one might take 400 neonates with meningomyelocele from among a group of university children's hospitals and compare them to a second reference group of 400 very young were children matched by age, who were referred to the same hospitals for management of severe trauma. The question of such a project is whether exposure of the mother to a particular garden herbicide during pregnancy might be associated with development of meningomyelocele. One would interview the mothers of both groups of children to determine the proportion with exposure in each group during the corresponding pregnancies. Suppose that 32% of the mothers of children with meningomyelocele report being exposed to the chemical herbicide, and that only 8% of the mothers of children with multiple trauma report such exposure. One would then conclude that children whose mothers were exposed to the herbicide are approximately 5.5 times as likely to be born with meningomyelocele. In statistical or epidemiologic terms one would say that the odds ratio is about 5.

In case-control research, if one obtains odds ratios that are high, say, 6, 11 or 20 (meaning that a target outcome is 6 times, 11 times or 20 times more likely to occur in the presence of a suspected risk factor as compared to the absence of the risk factor), one has evidence of association between the target outcome and the risk factor. The strength of the association, as reflected in the high odds ratios, would suggest but not prove causality of the risk factor with respect to the target outcome. Findings from case-control studies can seldom be taken as conclusive evidence of cause, no matter how high the odds ratios. Moreover, odds ratios from case-control studies are often in the order of only 1.3, 1.8 or about 2. In such cases (assuming that statistical significance has been attained), evidence of association can be invoked to draw causal inferences only at great peril. There are specific ground rules about diagnosing causality from association – the Hill criteria described previously in this paper, for instance.

The key disadvantages to the case-control method are vulnerability to bias and the difficulty in judicious choice of reference groups for comparison. Recall bias is a prominent difficulty. Information is often incomplete. The advantages include smaller numbers of patients and shorter follow-up resulting in more quickly available results. In the case of a rare disease or adverse drug reactions, the case-control method is often the only feasible way of evaluating association between the risk factor and a clinical outcome.

Bias and Observer Variation in Clinical and Epidemiological Research

The term *bias in research* does not denote prejudice or bigotry. It is a technical term used to indicate *systematic error,* as distinct from *random error.* Bias is present when results are systematically distorted by something extraneous and often not even suspected. As a very simple example, if height measurements of people were taken under circumstances in which the study subjects were inadvertently standing on a wooden plate 5 mm high, all the measurements of a sample of 400 people would be biased by 5 mm in the direction of greater height than should have been shown. Such bias would affect not only each observation but also the summary expressions (such as averages or means) for the 400 people. Discussed below are a few, of many, types of bias.

Suggestion Bias

When questions about symptoms or signs are put in a manner that requires *spontaneous* volunteering of the information from the respondents, the results in terms of frequencies (incidences or prevalences) are invariably lower than in circumstances in which respondents react to a *probe* made by the interviewer. For instance, the rates of arthritic and rheumatic symptoms are much lower in response to questions which read, “In the last 2 weeks was there anything wrong with your health?” compared to the frequency one obtains if the question is phrased, “In the last 2 weeks have you had morning stiffness in your back and joints?” or “Have you had swelling of any joints in your body?”or “Do you now have pain on movement of your joints?” or “In the last 2 weeks have you had limitation of movement of your joints?” Indeed, the directive probing approach resulted in a period prevalence of arthritic and rheumatic symptoms of an unselected population that was seven times higher than that measured using the spontaneous approach. All related projects and international comparisons indicate a high probability that the information emanating from spontaneous reports may be more valid, although spontaneous reporting is usually afflicted by underreporting.

Recall Span Bias

Recall span bias is a systematic error that arises when persons in a population are asked to remember certain categories or events during a span of time prior to the interview. That the validity of reported illnesses can be compromised by the selection of a given recall period has been shown empirically. Over the past 20 years, in fact, there has been much research into the question of which recall spans are appropriate, taking into account the memory of ordinary respondents for health events. Due to the results of this research, it is uncommon in survey research concerning health to elicit symptoms, diagnoses or other related phenomena in ambulatory settings (out of hospital) with recall spans of more than 2 weeks. The World Health Organization International Collaborative Study of Medical Care Utilization adheres to such criteria. The Canada Health Survey and the United States National Health Survey also respect these standards.

There are several important causes of compromised validity due to recall span bias: these include memory, salience of the episode to the respondent, social desirability of certain kinds of responses, and ego threat. As an example of memory, consider a situation in which respondents are asked to remember their diet in a particular month 6–12 months prior to the interview. They simply cannot and could not remember such information; no one can. An example of salience of an event is a major roadway accident resulting in permanent physical loss or impairment; contrast how salient and "memorable" such an event is with the salience of a coughing episode after swallowing a piece of food "the wrong way". Researchers have documented the tendency to report certain socially desirable behaviours, such as saving money, voting and possession of library cards. Social desirability encourages more complete reporting of hospitalizations for relatively unembarrassing diseases, such as gallbladder surgery, than those for mental and personality disorders. Underreporting as a result of ego threat occurs when people deny the occurrence of an event because it is very threatening to them; this is why cancer is regularly underreported in surveys, and also why abnormal reproductive events, including birth defects, are underreported.

Interviewer Bias

The potential for interviewers to bias data is well known. There is much evidence that respondents report and/or interviewers record information based on their own expectations of each other. Hence, standardization of interviewer appearance through intensive training in dress, probes and non-judgmental attitudes, and blinding to the study purpose have become standard practice. Interviewer bias may result from the interviewer's perception of the respondent, the respondent's assessment of the interviewer's attitudes and expectations, or from both of these sources. For example, working class interviewers report more radical political attitudes among their respondents than do "middle-class" interviewers, and blacks are more apt to report racism to non-whites than to whites.

Respondent Bias

The respondent filters his response through his own beliefs, attitudes and goals. Perception is often distorted by personal experience. For example, a woman who cannot conceive may be more likely than other women to notice "how many women she knows who are pregnant". Similarly, once a contaminated landfill is discovered nearby, symptoms which might have been present before the respondent moved to that area might acquire new significance for that respondent.

Observer Bias or Observer Variability

It is a frequent observation in clinical studies that measurements by clinicians, particularly doctors, vary from one instance to another with the same patient or between doctors on the same patient to such an extent that sometimes the reproducibility between measurements is barely better than that which would be observed by chance. Clinicians and particularly doctors making measurements or assessments for research purposes must be very rigorously trained, almost "decerebrated", to do ritualized examinations so that observer variation can be brought to a minimum, and so that clinical findings used in population studies can be used with any measure of confidence as to their reliability.

Conclusion

Evaluating evidence that establishes effectiveness, safety, risk, harm and other attributes of therapies and health interventions requires a reasonable understanding of design, measurement, bias and principles of causality. There are certain rules of admissibility for scientific evidence which must be respected if research data are to be used appropriately in decisions about drugs and health. Evaluation of published evidence should take such rules into account, reinforced by strong doses of clinical judgement, statistical knowledge and, above all, common sense.

Adapted in part from: Spitzer WO (1986) Selected non-experimental methods: an orientation. In: Troidl H, Spitzer WO, McPeek B, Mulder DS, McKneally MS (eds) Principles and practices of research: strategies for surgical investigators, 1st edn. Springer, Berlin Heidelberg New York (Sect. III Chap. 8)

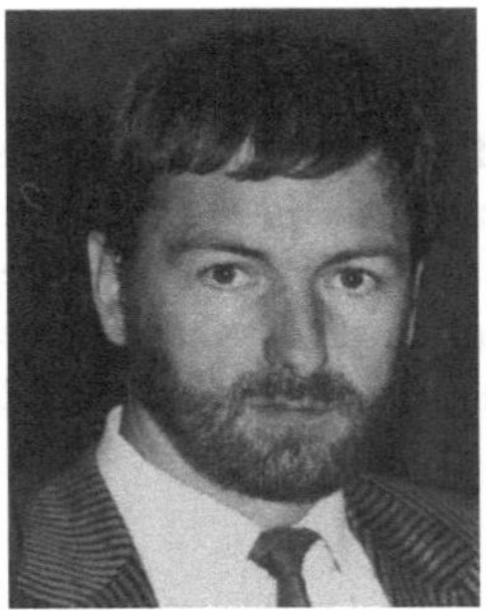

8. Statistics in Drug Risk Research: The Background of Pharmacoepidemiology

H. LETZEL

Risk Perception and Statistics

Public, political and scientific concerns about drug safety or drug risk are embedded in a wider spectrum of "low-risk" perception and management, whether it be a dam, lung cancer from passive smoking, health hazards from low-dose radiation or similar risk sources. To some extent the perception of risk depends on whether a manifestation of the risk has already taken place or not. Thalidomide and Chernobyl have clearly shown this. They also show that *low* risk refers only to the likelihood, not the severity, of an adverse event. The term seems to mask the fact that risk may be low but is nevertheless present, and the consequences may range from small to immeasurable. "Low risk" gives rise to the illusion that nothing deleterious will in fact happen.

Thus, risk perception plays a great role in risk management. The role of statistics is to add a rational element to expectation. Historically, statistics has been a mathematical theory of gambling. Some people have always had a tendency to gamble regardless of the odds because they believe in their chances, particularly if a substantial amount of money is at stake. They are not surprised if they win, because they gambled thinking a priori that they would have a chance. The actual likelihood of winning is not considered.[1]

Using drugs is different. People take them because they weigh likelihoods completely differently. The likelihood of dying from taking aspirin may be on the same order of magnitude as winning the lottery game. So to some extent the whole benefit/risk discussion – regardless of which topic it is applied to – is primarily a psychological or, in other words, an emotional problem. It is no surprise, therefore, that accidents are not evaluated according to their respective likelihood to cause harm but rather by the amount of harm caused once manifestation has taken place – regardless as to how unlikely it was that this would happen. Thalidomide was the turning point regarding

[1] In a lottery game "6 out of 49", which is very popular in the Federal Republic of Germany, the odds are given by the binomial coefficient:

$$\binom{n}{k} = \binom{49}{6} = \frac{49 \times 48 \times \ldots \times 44}{1 \times 2 \times \ldots \times 6}$$

The likelihood of guessing correctly is, therefore, 1 : 13983816

drug safety, comparable to the Chernobyl disaster in questioning the use of nuclear power.

One decisive tool for effective risk management has been seen during the past few decades in the application of statistical methods to clinical and epidemiological research. The basic concepts as well as the basic limitations of the statistical approach towards drug risk research are examined in this article. After bias and confounding, which are covered in the presentation by Spitzer, the third fundamental limitation is the question of whether the sample size required statistically can be realized. Some aspects of sample size calculations are, therefore, included.

Statistical Concepts for the Discovery of Drug Risk

Risk assessment always includes two questions: Is there an increase in risk? and How large is this risk? The attempt to answer these questions can follow two different directions, the comparative approach or the non-comparative approach.

Comparative approach

The fundamental feature of the comparative approach is that two or more groups of persons under risk (i.e. taking certain drugs or placebo) are compared. If this is done in a prospective mode with randomized allocation to treatment groups, it is called a controlled clinical trial. If it is done retrospectively, it is called a case-control study.

Controlled Clinical Trials. The well-known basic model (Fig. 8.1) compares the relative frequencies P_1 and P_2 of adverse events between the treatment groups by means of a χ^2 test:

$$\chi^2 = \frac{(a\,d - b\,c)^2\,n}{(a + b)\,(a + c)\,(b + d)\,(c + d)}$$

With one degree of freedom the critical values of the χ^2 distribution which must be surmounted are 3.841 for $p \leq 0.05$, or 6.635 for $p \leq 0.01$, respectively.

		Adverse Experience: Yes	Adverse Experience: No	
Drug	A	a	b	$P_1 = \frac{a}{a+b}$
	B	c	d	$P_2 = \frac{c}{c+d}$

Fig. 8.1. A 2 × 2 table for comparison of the frequency of adverse events between two treatment groups

This model has been successfully used in efficacy studies. However, it has serious limitations in drug risk research for rare events because the χ^2 test requires a considerable sample size in order to detect small differences between two treatment groups. If more than two treatment groups are to be compared, the number of patients required increases even more. A practical recommendation is, therefore, that clinical trials should in most cases be restricted to comparing two groups. This is particularly so in the case of safety studies. Blinding is mandatory if the assessment of the effects under study can be affected by observation bias.

For the planning of such studies a sample size estimation should be performed. A formula commonly used for this is:

$$n = \left(\frac{z_{\alpha/2} \sqrt{2\bar{p}\bar{q}} + z_\beta \sqrt{p_1 q_1 + p_2 q_2}}{|D|} \right)^2 + \frac{2}{|D|}$$

The following variables can be derived from Fig. 8.1:

$\bar{p} = (P_1 + P_2) : 2$
$\bar{q} = ((1 - P_1) + (1 - P_2)) : 2$
$p_1 = P_1$
$p_2 = P_2$
$q_1 = (1 - P_1)$
$q_2 = (1 - P_2)$
$D = P_1 - P_2$

Using this formula, examples were calculated for a scenario in which it was assumed that a standard drug B would lead to certain side effects with a likelihood of P_2 = 2%–5%, whereas a new drug A could reduce this rate to $P_1 = 1\%$. The likelihood of detecting such a difference if it exists is called "power". Table 8.1 shows that the comparison between side effects occurring in 1% versus 2% of patients can require up to 3300 patients per group. This figure can be reduced by a compromise in power. For efficacy studies investigators are often satisfied with a power of 0.8. Therefore, corresponding calculations are included in Table 8.1.

There is no strict rule as to what the power should be, but there is a clear-cut line below which a study does not make any sense. This is a power of 50% (third row in Table 8.1). At this power the likelihood of finding a difference, if it exists, as a result of a study is equivalent to the likelihood of coming to the right conclusion as the result of tossing a coin – in addition to the fact that a study would waste time and money and would have to include up to 1328 patients per group.

Table 8.1. Sample sizes required to establish statistical significance by a χ^2 test of a 2 × 2 table at the 5% level for side effects occurring in 1% (P_1) versus 2%–5% (P_2)

	P_2			
Power	0.02	0.03	0.04	0.05
0.9	3300	1125	632	429
0.8	2514	865	488	332
0.5	1328	471	271	186

$P_1 = 0.01$, $\alpha = 0.05$

This shows, in summary, that single controlled clinical trials are very unlikely to reveal differences in drug risk between treatment groups. It remains to be seen to what extent this situation could be improved by meta-analysis, i.e. the statistical pooling of results obtained by several studies.

Case-Control Studies. One of the ideas underlying a case-control study is to get around the sample size hurdle discussed in the preceding paragraphs. The only reason that a large sample size is necessary for risk comparisons between two treatment groups is the rareness of the event. So why not omit observing all those patients who do not develop the side effect? The resulting (retrospective) study design is called a case-control study (for details see the chapter by Spitzer in this volume). The price to be paid for the gain in sample size reduction and the saving of time and money can be validity. By the time the study starts, everything has already happened: persons have or have not been exposed to a certain drug, and the event under study has already occurred. It could even be that a patient does not exist any more because he has died in the meantime.

For sample size estimates the above formula for a 2 × 2 design can be adapted. Depending on the magnitude of the assumed relative risk, up to a few hundred patients must be included per group. If the relative risk is marked, less than 100 cases per group may be sufficient to reach statistical significance. The discussion on suitable sample sizes, however, should not mask the fact that the main methodological problem of a case-control study is the minimization of bias and confounding.

In summary, case-control studies are in many instances the only method to assess causality between a suspect drug and a postulated noxious effect. Their use should, therefore, be encouraged. But even more: their methodology should be developed further.

Non-comparative Approach

The aim of the non-comparative approach is detecting and quantifying adverse drug effects. It includes spontaneous reports and observational studies. Spontaneous reports are normally the source from which hypotheses about rare new side effects are first generated, but they are not suitable for corroborating or refuting hypotheses. Neither can observational studies prove causal conclusions, but in contrast to spontaneous reports they sometimes allow the determination of the frequency with which a side effect must be encountered.

Phase IV studies with large sample sizes but no control groups are frequently used in order to establish more data on drug safety. This approach basically seems to make sense since during the pre-registration period rarely more than a few thousand patients are included in clinical trials of a new compound. This means that our knowledge of rare side effects is bound to be limited at the time of registration.

The more successful, rapid market penetration strategies are, the more patients will be treated with the new drug within a very short period of time – and sometimes without sufficiently close supervision. This is certainly one of the most dangerous periods in the "life" of a drug. If the drug causes rare side effects, these happen suddenly, and there is a variable time lag until the course is identified, and appropriate steps are taken. Quite a few very effective drugs have been withdrawn from the market soon after successful seeding. It is a matter of speculation how many of them could still be on the market if there had been more time to learn about and to deal with new side effects step by step.

From a probabilistic point of view, the question could be formulated: "How many patients receiving the new drug must be monitored in order to detect at least one patient with a side effect that occurs with a probability (p) if one wants to be sure with a certain power (P) not to miss this side effect?"

In order to answer this question a binomial distribution is commonly used. It leads to a simple equation for the number of cases required:

$$n = \frac{ln\,(1-P)}{ln\,(1-p)}$$

A scenario of various sample sizes which were calculated by this formula is given in Table 8.2. This table shows that for a certain frequency of a side effect (e.g. 1 in 10000, equivalent to $p = 0.01$) roughly three times as many patients (i.e. 29956) must be monitored if at least one occurrence of the side effect is to be detected with a power of $P = 95\%$. It is a philosophical question whether an incidence of 1 in 10000 for a severe or even fatal side effect represents a rare or a frequent event. This depends on the prognosis of the underlying disease, alternative treatment and other factors. But the calculations show that many post-marketing drug surveillance studies have a low chance of detecting such an event.

Table 8.2. Number of patients needed to observe at least one patient with a side effect

	Probability of side effect (p)		
Power (P)	0.01	0.005	0.001
0.95	29956	59914	229572
0.80	16094	32188	160943
0.50	6932	13863	69315

For the strategic planning of sample sizes an assumed power of 50% is a good reference line. This calculation uses the number of patients (i.e. 6932) necessary for a study which has a likelihood of observing at least one case with a side effect that occurs once in 10000 patients – and is about the same likelihood as the result of tossing a coin.

In summary, these calculations show that the chances of detecting rare and as yet unknown side effects of drugs in observational studies are limited even with relatively large sample sizes.

The situation becomes even worse when three fundamental pitfalls of the underlying model are taken into account. In the above calculations it was assumed that (a) all patients treated have an equal likelihood of developing an adverse event; (b) every single event will be observed and correctly linked to the given drug; and (c) the duration of treatment and/or observation has no influence. For methods of simplicity we only look at the second point and introduce the "3 × 50% rule". This rule assumes: (a) 50% of the occurring adverse events will be observed; (b) 50% of the

Table 8.3. Loss of power due to failures in observing, linking and reporting adverse events: the resulting power in relation to the original power and the three levels of the "3 × 50% rule"

p	Original power	1 × 50% (2 events)	2 × 50% (4 events)	3 × 50% (8 events)
0.05	0.95	0.80	0.35	0.008
	0.80	0.48	0.07	0.0001
	0.50	0.15	0.004	< 0.0001
0.001	0.95	0.80	0.35	0.012
	0.80	0.48	0.08	0.0003
	0.50	0.15	0.006	< 0.0001

observed adverse events will be correctly linked to the drug given; and (c) 50% of these adverse events correctly linked to the drug will be reported. This means that the number of events that must occur doubles on each of these three levels. Using the scenario of Table 8.2, eight events actually must occur until the first report will be made. This leads to an enormous loss of power, which is shown in Table 8.3.

Figures from Table 8.2 were used for the calculations in Table 8.3. In summary, the introduction of the "3 × 50% rule" – which can be regarded as a very conservative, if not even over-optimistic view of clinical research – leads to sample size calculations which can completely destroy all rational hope of detecting rare side effects of drugs in observational studies.

Discussion

In this paper we have examined sample size calculations for comparative and non-comparative study designs for clinical and epidemiological drug risk research. We have seen that the systematic investigation of rare adverse events is questioned by the enormous sample sizes that may be required. This situation points to a fact and raises a question.

The *fact*: If the power of observational studies is too low, even at sample sizes of a few ten thousand patients, then we really rely on spontaneous case reports of doctors observing adverse events during and/or after the prescription of a drug. In order to elicit such spontaneous reports the majority of doctors need a better understanding of pharmacoepidemiology.

The *question*: Are there other relevant factors that can be studied to improve drug safety? The answer is yes. There are at least two constituents of drug risk – intrinsic and extrinsic factors or the properties of the drug versus the way we use it. So far, we have concentrated primarily on the intrinsic factor, i.e. the pharmaceutical and pharmacological properties of the drug. We have thought that they are the primary constituents of drug risk, and that they can be successfully investigated by qualified pharmaceutical expertise as well as by qualified pharmacological, clinical and epidemiological research. But we have not taken the extrinsic factor seriously enough, i.e. how a drug is used by a doctor and his patient.

In the above paragraphs we have come to the conclusion that clinical studies have severe limitations regarding the discovery of drug risk. We have also seen that with these tools we cannot investigate how doctors (and patients) use registered drugs under everyday conditions. We should, therefore, study these phenomena which constitute the extrinsic factor of drug risk. With regard to the doctor, there are at least two dimensions. The first dimension is the doctor's experience – with the specific drug and its alternatives, with the disease(s) to be treated with this drug, and with the patient for whom the drug is prescribed.

At present I feel that the investigation of this dimension should best be left to medical quality control programmes. The other dimension is the actual behaviour of the doctor: for *whom* he prescribes *what* drug in *what* dose in *which* situation (concomitant disease(s) and medication, extra-medical frame) for *how* long. But this dimension also includes the doctor's interaction with his patient during follow-up.

On the patient's side, we should consider his intelligence and awareness, his attitude towards suffering symptoms and taking drugs, his self-medication as well as his eating and drinking and other personal habits, his reporting behaviour to his doctors and his overall attitude towards benifits and risks of illness and medical therapy. We know very little about these factors. The work by Slovic described in this volume is one of the first approaches to study the patient more closely. Further work will have to follow. This should include surveys on patients suffering from certain diseases or taking certain drugs. But on top of this, particular emphasis will have to be put on learning more about the doctors' approaches to drug therapy. The existing technology of computers and telecommunications offers promising ways of linking general practices via computer networks to central statistical units which collect prescription data, feed them back to the prescriber and assist him via expert systems in making the right decisions. We should move in this direction.

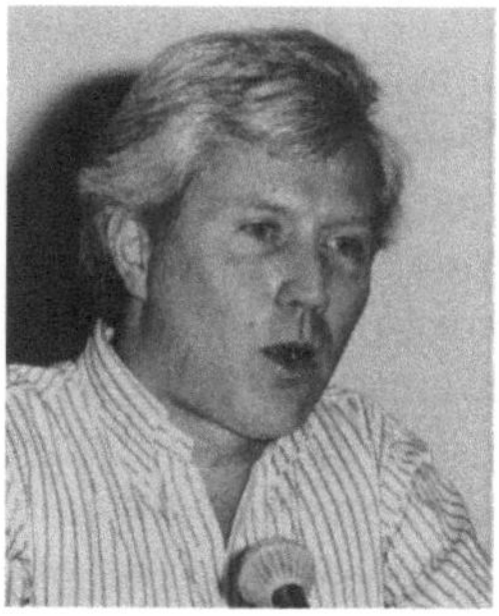

9. Industry-Sponsored Risk Institutes

W. W. Lowrance

From time to time it has been proposed that the international pharmaceutical enterprise, perhaps including other organizations along with corporations, consider establishing one or more semiautonomous institutes to conduct analyses and convene forums on a variety of generic, nonproprietary issues. In analogous enterprises (such as those described below), institutes of this kind render substantial public service.

The purpose of this presentation is to outline the characteristics of some risk institutes that have been successfully established in the United States and to suggest how institutes of this kind might be useful in the pharmaceutical arena.

A certain reservation should be expressed at the outset, however. From deep in the human psyche there seems to arise, whenever a social problem becomes identified, a reflex to form an institute. Indeed, I have helped build a few myself. But surely we should hold a tentative presumption against forming new institutions unless they genuinely offer promise for accomplishing novel and sound objectives.

Some Illuminating Examples

The following vignettes describe institutes that have made firm contributions to the understanding and management of health and environmental risk issues. All of them are predominantly sponsored by American industrial firms. A few have sponsors or members from outside the United States. Several are funded by governmental or philanthropic sources in addition to corporations.

Chemical Industry Institute of Technology (CIIT). Supported by 35 large chemical companies. Founded 1975. Budget in fiscal year 1986 U.S. $13000000. Mixed member-company and outsider Board of Directors, complemented by an external Scientific Advisory Panel. CIIT is a substantial, free-standing, innovative laboratory that pursues fundamental toxicological research on heavy nonproprietary chemicals, such as solvents. It also evaluates methods, provides postdoctoral training, and holds scientific conferences. Its primary purpose is to develop the field of chemical toxicology.

Health Effects Institute (HEI). Jointly sponsored by a group of 26 automotive manufacturers and the United States Environmental Protection Agency (50%/50% funding). Founded 1980. Budget 1986 \$7000000. Independent Board of Directors sets overall goals; an autonomous nonindustry Research Committee develops and awards research contracts; a similar but separate Review Committee critiques the scientific merit and risk-assessment relevance of the resulting research products. HEI awards external research contracts to a variety of universities, consulting firms, and other organizations to investigate health effects from motor vehicle emissions. In its initial years, it concentrated on diesel emission effects. Soon HEI will complete an elaborate Future Strategy Project charting the research needs of the 1990s. One product of this project is the 1988 book, *Air Pollution, the Automobile, and Public Health* (National Academy Press, Washington, DC).

Center for Chemical Process Safety (CCPS). Established in the aftermath of the Bhopal disaster in India, as a directorate of the American Institute of Chemical Engineers (the professional society). Founded 1985. Supported by some 50 corporations and foundations. Budget 1986 \$600000. Diversified Managing Board and Advisory Board. CCPS develops and evaluates technical and operational practices to predict, prevent, and mitigate major accidental releases of toxic chemicals. It also publishes practical guidelines on such topics as hazard evaluation and vapor-release mitigation.

Electric Power Research Institute (EPRI). Supported by 562 member utilities. Founded 1973. Budget 1986 \$306000000 (a portion of which is devoted to risks). Industry Board of Directors and outside Advisory Council. EPRI conducts a wide range of technological research and development, and it studies a variety of health and environmental risk issues relating to electric power generation and delivery. Recent major projects have focused, for example, on acid rain and on health effects from very low level chronic exposure to the electromagnetic fields that surround powerlines. Currently the Institute supervises some 1500 research projects (again, only some are on risk problems) in a variety of institutions around the world. It also develops methods and holds technical conferences.

Risk Science Institute (RSI) of the International Life Sciences Institute. Supported by 120 food, chemical, and pharmaceutical companies. Founded 1985. Budget 1987 \$1000000. RSI commissions extramural research and holds conferences on scientific risk assessment issues, such as interspecies metabolic comparisons and evaluation of statistical methods.

Other Trade Institutes. Several other industry organizations sponsor, among other things, risk-related research and assessment. Examples are the American Petroleum Institute and the Gas Research Institute. In general, institutes of this kind provide service to trade members. They may or may not take elaborate measures to publish their work, involve outsiders, or cultivate external credibility.

The (Former) Food Safety Council. This organization, a nonprofit consortium of food companies and a variety of other groups, worked hard in the late 1970s to develop guidelines for food risk analysis and policy. The scientific part succeeded and produced an influential report, but the policy part experienced great difficulty in developing consensus. Perhaps lessons could be gleaned by reviewing the historical dynamics of this endeavor.

Scope of Coverage

A key question is whether an organization of this kind should address technical problems, ethical-political-economic problems, or a combination. This choice should be addressed deliberately, and should be expressed in the institution's charter. A purely technical institute should fiercely protect its work against nontechnical politization, and it should incorporate all appropriate mechanisms of scientific peer review. A more political institute should be candid about the sociopolitical nature of its program and should expect to become involved in controversial social exchanges. The institution should be structured in accordance with whatever scope is chosen.

A related question is whether an institute should mainly provide service to the sponsors, or whether it should reach for broader stewardship, such as educating journalists or building societal consensus on issues. Again, this choice has implications for structure.

Organizational Characteristics

For any such institute, organizational determinants of quality and social legitimacy include:

A diverse, worldly, active board of directors.
A competent professional staff.
Insulation of programs, once committed to, from ad hoc meddling by individual sponsoring firms.
Stable financing from multiple sources.
Firm separation of "risk" activities from industry promotional activities.
Independent critical evaluation of quality and relevance of accomplishments.
Strategic medium-term focusing on issues of broad concern.
Good-faith public outreach.

Existing Pharmaceutical Institutes

Several institutes already exist that work on pharmaceutical issues, of course. These include, for example, the Center for the Study of Drug Development at Tufts University in Boston, the Boston Collaborative Drug Surveillance Program, the Drug Safety Research Unit at Southampton University in Sussex, and the Centre for Medicines Research in Surrey. In this conference we have learned of a new Institute for Medicines Monitoring in the United Kingdom. And there are others. Some of these organizations might well expand their agendas to include risk work or to extend over a broader range of risk concerns. Several of them have the inherent shortcoming of dealing with risk issues even as they promote drug development and use. In any event, they should be held to the standards listed above, just as a new institute should.

Some Possible Functions

A variety of functions can be performed by risk institutes. The following, ordered roughly from the technical to the political, indicate the range of possibilities.

First, an institute might pursue rather fundamental research on scientific themes of generic interest. Probably it should avoid working extensively on individual proprietary products, except as case examples or as part of clusters of products from several manufacturers. An example of such a theme might be the dynamics of accumulation of drugs and drug metabolites in amniotic fluid.

Second, it might pursue practical problem solving. A few years ago such a center could have conducted or coordinated research and development on tamper-resistant packaging. At present, it might beneficially scrutinize technical and regulatory issues surrounding drug delivery devices.

Third, it might innovate, revise, or evaluate the technical procedures and methods, such as adverse-reaction reporting mechanisms or pharmacoepidemiology, that comprise the factual foundation upon which the entire industry is built.

Fourth, it might evaluate how scientific analyses are used in managerial and regulatory decision making, and how criteria are developed for deciding whether a drug's risks are acceptable under given clinical circumstances.

Fifth, it might review, certify, and endorse various risk-assessment, risk/benefit, cost-effectiveness, or other analyses to government bodies and the public. This would have to be done extremely carefully to assure the highest quality and credibility of review and avoid undue bias – and appearance of bias.

Sixth, it might work to educate health care providers, journalists, special patient groups, and the general public as to the proper use of drugs, the nature of pharmaceutical decisions, and the shape of the pharmaceutical enterprise. In this regard it might also help improve the usefulness of physician and patient-package informational materials.

And seventh, it might play a variety of quite public roles, such as convening stocktaking or consensus forums on controversial topical issues.

Conclusion

On some of these efforts, industry-sponsored institutes might work alone effectively. On others, they might work better in concert with traditional academic research centers. On the most sociopolitical, they might work best in coalitions with advocacy groups, professional societies, government agencies, or intergovernmental bodies.

The most important characteristics of any such institute are: (a) the highest possible quality of analytic work; (b) social credibility of the organization and its leadership; and (c) broad, sustained advancement of the basic enterprise.

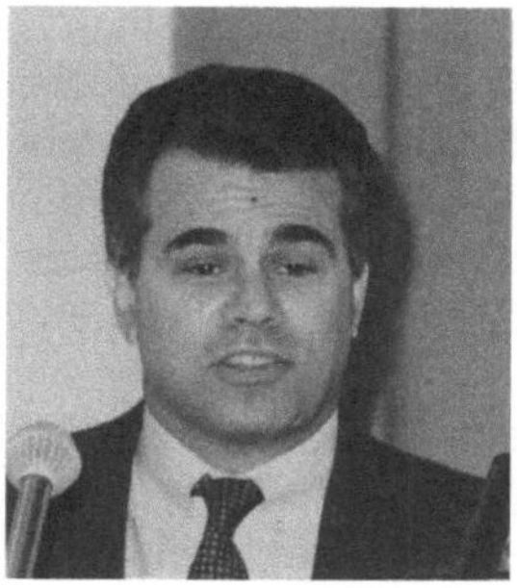

10. The Feldene Experience: A Case Study

R. M. SACHS, G. S. DIECK

Introduction

The following illustrates an actual experience involving allegations of safety problems with the nonsteroidal anti-inflammatory drug (NSAID) Feldene (piroxicam). It is intended to serve as a case study of the ramifications of examining complex issues of risk analysis in a public forum under volatile conditions. Although the safety of the drug was ultimately established, both the process and its conclusion had significant impact on the manufacturer, the regulatory agency, physicians and patients. This discussion will focus particularly on the roles played in this episode by pharmacoepidemiology and the media.

Chronology

In April 1982, piroxicam was approved in the United States. It received wide-spread usage, and rapidly became one of the most widely prescribed NSAIDs in the United States. In July 1982 a Congressional Oversight Committee hearing was held dealing primarily with the safety of another NSAID, benoxaprofen, which was removed from the market shortly thereafter under controversial conditions. Although piroxicam was briefly considered at that hearing, no major safety issues were raised. Approximately 1 year later, the Bundesgesundheitsamt (BGA), the West German regulatory body, expressed concern about the safety of piroxicam. A hearing on piroxicam was held, but no significant safety problems were found.

The Arthritis Advisory Committee of the United States Food and Drug Administration (FDA) met in October 1984 [1]. At that meeting the FDA presented summary tables of spontaneously reported adverse reactions for each NSAID with denominator values derived from estimates of the number of prescriptions written within a specified time period. The initial goal of the FDA was to use these tables as a basis for comparing the safety of the various NSAIDs, but after the limitations of using spontaneous reports for causality assessments were discussed, the Advisory Committee rejected the tables as unacceptable for use as a basis for comparison of drug safety. The issue was again raised at the next Arthritis Advisory Committee meeting in April 1985, and the Advisory Committee again concluded that spontaneous report data were not an appropriate basis for this type of regulatory action [2].

In December 1985 a British newspaper, *The Observer,* published an article citing 77 deaths reportedly related to piroxicam, based upon information obtained from uncorrected registry figures [3]. Shortly thereafter, in January 1986, the Health Research Group (HRG), a consumer activist group based in the United States, filed a petition to the Department of Health and Human Services (HHS), requesting that piroxicam be declared an "imminent hazard," and that its use in the United States be severely restricted [4].

After the petition was filed on January 8, 1986, HHS referred the matter to the FDA which scheduled a hearing on February 28 [5]. The Docket (a special file set up by FDA to contain all documents pertaining to the petition) was kept open until March 17 for the filing of additional pertinent information by any interested party. On July 7, 1986, the petition was formally denied [6].

Magnitude of the Response

The HRG petition itself was an 11-page letter. It was denied in a two-page letter from HHS Secretary Bowen [6]. In the 6 months which intervened between these two rather short documents, HRG submitted an additional 10-page letter to the Docket with corresponding references, and an enormous effort was put forth by both Pfizer Inc. and the FDA to accumulate and evaluate piroxicam safety data. Pfizer's response consisted of a 12-page letter plus four volumes (nearly 700 total pages) of analysis, supported by six volumes of reference materials [7]. The FDA, after analyzing the Pfizer submission, responded with a 60-page analysis [8] which was summarized in a seven-page memo from the Commissioner of the FDA to the Secretary of HHS [9].

The relative volume of material generated by the various parties is instructive, but the content of these documents is of greater importance.

HRG Petition

The core of the HRG petition was the spontaneously reported adverse-event data generated by the FDA. The spontaneous or anecdotal reporting system, although useful as a signalling device, is known to have significant limitations with regard to quantitative or comparative use. These limitations have been discussed in detail elsewhere [10] and will be considered here only briefly.

A major characteristic of spontaneous report data is that drugs typically have their peak of adverse reaction reporting during the first 2 years that the product is on the market. Subsequently, the number of reports declines. This is sometimes referred to as the Weber curve [11]. In addition to the effects on the reporting of spontaneous events described by the Weber curve, reporting is also a function of secular changes in reporting habits such as those that may be caused by publicity surrounding a drug or drug class or changes in reporting systems.

Piroxicam entered the United States market in 1982, when all reports of spontaneous events to the FDA were rapidly increasing [12] (Table 10.1). Figure 10.1 illustrates the variability of ADR reports by calendar year and by year since launch. In 1980, substantially more ADRs were reported for Clinoril than for other NSAIDs. In

Table 10.1. Total spontaneous ADR reports submitted to FDA (1981–1985)

1981	15000
1982	28600
1983	35000
1984	36000
1985	45700

Source: FDA Division of Epidemiology

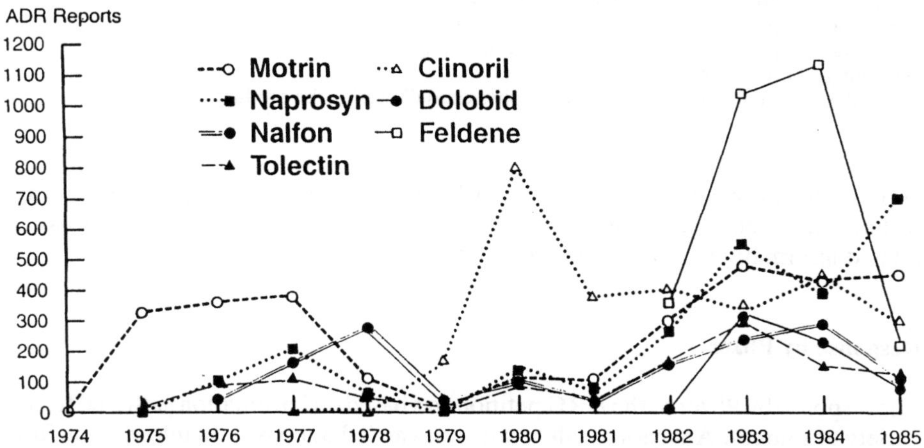

Fig. 10.1. ADR reports by calendar year. From 1986 FDA Spontaneous Reporting System, printout February 14, 1986

1983, the highest number of ADRs was found for Feldene; however, in 1985 Naprosyn had the highest number of reports while both Feldene and Clinoril had considerably less. Thus, misleading conclusions may be reached by taking a cross-sectional approach to ADR reporting. Even after accounting for differences according to both secular and marketing trends, what remains is at best a corrected signal.

Another factor that may affect the safety profile of a drug compared to others in its therapeutic class is how and to whom the drug is administered. In the United States, different NSAIDs are prescribed for different reasons to different subgroups of the population. For instance, as seen in Table 10.2, some drugs are prescribed for long courses for chronic conditions while others are prescribed for acute conditions, and exposure may be for a matter of hours or days. Some drugs are prescribed primarily for arthritis, such as Feldene and Clinoril, while others (Motrin and Dolobid) are generally used for analgesia, as in sprains or strains. Clinoril and Feldene are more likely to be prescribed for individuals over age 60, while Motrin and Dolobid are commonly prescribed for those aged under 60 years. Indocin is less likely to be given to women than are other nonsteroidals. Detailing time, sales representatives' interaction with physicians, is a major source of adverse reporting. Consequently, the more active detailing to which newer drugs are generally subject, may provide greater

Table 10.2. Profiles of five NSAIDs in the United States (1984)

	Piroxicam	Clinoril	Motrin	Indocin	Dolobid
Years on market	2	6	10	19	2
Days therapy/prescription	26	25	16	19	14
[1]Rx for arthritis (%)	78	71	49	57	18
[2]Patients over 60 years of age (%)	56	51	39	45	34
[3]Patients under 40 years of age (%)	11	21	34	23	36
[4]Women (%)	68	66	66	51	64
[5]Detail time (millions of min)	1.6	0.9	1.4	0.6	1.2

[1]Percentage of prescriptions used for treatment of arthritis.
[2]Percentage of prescriptions used for patients over age 60.
[3]Percentage of prescriptions used for patients under age 40.
[4]Percentage of prescriptions used for women.
[5]Time the sales representatives spend with physicians discussing the product.

opportunity for events to be reported. Clearly, direct comparisons between drugs within a therapeutic class may be misleading unless some of these usage patterns and related information are taken into account.

Response by Pfizer

The response by Pfizer to the HRG petition was based on information gathered from a variety of sources. Analysis of safety data was carried out based on information from over 5000 patients from 68 comparative clinical trials [13]. Additional postmarketing surveillance data on over 50000 patients worldwide were also evaluated. Nine formal epidemiologic studies were introduced in support of piroxicam's relative safety, the details of which will be discussed below [14]. Finally, the results of 11 pharmacokinetic studies were presented in response to a separate issue that had been raised. Despite the variety of information provided and reviewed, pharmacoepidemiology was the basis for the critical information upon which the decision was made to deny the petition.

When reports surfaced in late 1985 about gastrointestinal bleeding among patients who took Pfizer Inc.'s anti-arthritis drug piroxicam, "we called everybody in" who had medical-record data bases to help investigate, says Gerald Faich, who directs the FDA division that monitors adverse drug reactions. "Much of the data we used" in deciding no actions were needed in the matter came from their studies, he adds [15].

Epidemiologic Studies

Epidemiologic studies were commissioned by both Pfizer and the FDA. As is characteristic of epidemiologists, most current findings and study results were shared with Pfizer, the FDA, and HRG, regardless of who sponsored the research. Analyses were carried out by Jick at the Boston Collaborative Drug Surveillance Program (BCDSP) [16], Strom of the University of Pennsylvania who used Michigan Medicaid data [17], and by Ray of Vanderbilt University who examined Tennessee Medicaid data [18]. A fourth study, carried out by Inman in the United Kingdom, used the prescription event monitoring (PEM) system set up in that country [19]. These four studies were cohort studies. The BCDSP and Michigan Medicaid studies were designed to examine upper gastrointestinal bleeding (in hospitalized patients only for the BCDSP), while the PEM study also considered perforation. The Tennessee Medicaid Study examined deaths due to upper gastrointestinal disorders only.

In addition to the cohort studies, observational epidemiologic studies using a case-control design were also carried out. The study by Shapiro of the Slone Epidemiology Unit examined upper gastrointestinal bleeding among hospitalized patients using data from the United States, Canada, and Israel [20]. A separate study by Somerville in the United Kingdom focused on bleeding peptic ulcers among hospitalized patients [21].

Finally, three case review studies provided support; the investigators of these three reviews also had access to local data on nonsteroidal use so that a rough denominator figure was available. Among hospitalized patients these reviews examined upper gastrointestinal bleeding [22], upper gastrointestinal bleeding and perforation [23], and bleeding peptic ulcer [24]. A brief summary of the results of nine studies using three basic design strategies is found in Table 10.3.

Table 10.3. Result of observational studies

		Study conclusions			
Researchers	Method	NSAID risk?	ASA risk NSAID risk?	NSAID difference?	Feldene difference?
Inman	Cohort	No	NT[a]	No	No
Jick	Cohort	No	NT	No	No
Strom	Cohort	Yes	NT	Yes	No
Ray	Cohort	?	NT	Yes	No
Somerville	Case-control	Yes	NT	NT	NT
Shapiro	Case-control	Yes	Yes	NT	NT
Haglund	Case review	Yes	Yes	NT	NT
Giercksky	Case review	NT	Yes	No	No
O'Brien	Case review	NT	NT	?	No

[a] NT, not tested

Findings were generally consistent, but not uniform. Two cohort studies reported no detectable increased risk associated with NSAID use, four studies using all three study designs reported that use of NSAIDs was associated with an increased risk. Two case reviews did not examine the issue, and one cohort study had insufficient data. Only three studies examined the risk of gastrointestinal disorder with aspirin use compared to other NSAIDs, and all three reported a higher risk with aspirin. Of the five studies that examined differences between NSAIDs, three reported that no differences were detectable, while two reported differences but were not consistent with each other. The four cohort studies were split evenly on this issue. The most consistent finding was that of the six studies that examined piroxicam specifically; none reported a significant increase in risk for users of piroxicam compared to other NSAIDs. The consistency of this latter finding was one basis for the subsequent denial of the HRG "imminent hazard" petition.

Regulatory Result

The premise on which the HRG petition was based was that "GI toxicity is more common and severe with Feldene than with similar arthritis drugs, particularly in elderly patients [4]." However, the FDA and the Department of HHS reached a different conclusion. The FDA stated in its 60-page analysis, that "of available epidemiologic data and published and unpublished retrospective case analyses ... no basis for concluding that piroxicam is more likely to cause serious gastrointestinal toxicity in the elderly than similar products" was found [8]. Epidemiologic evidence was cited as the basis for these conclusions. The FDA further noted that "in citing the spontaneous reports, the HRG ignored the rudimentary precautions needed to evaluate such data" and, in fact, "ignored the well-known limitations, presenting wholly unadjusted data [8]." Although pharmacokinetic considerations were raised, the FDA concluded that "... in the absence of sound epidemiologic or clinical trial data that piroxicam does ... pose a greater risk ..., the pharmacokinetic considerations became irrelevant to the question of imminent hazard [8]." Perhaps the most significant conclusion by the FDA stated, "Because properly analyzed epidemiologic and spontaneous report data fail to provide evidence of an excess of G.I. toxicity with piroxicam, ... data from controlled clinical trials ... is not critical to a decision [9]." By such statements the FDA endorsed the use of pharmacoepidemiology as a major tool in assessing drug safety.

Costs

Although Pfizer had the means and ability to respond, it is worth considering that smaller companies might not have the same resources to devote to such an effort. It is estimated that at least 80 in-house personnel and well over a million dollars were devoted to the defense. The petition was also costly to the FDA with respect to time and money. As of June 9, 1986, over 246 person-days, much of it senior staff time, and about $ 50000 had been spent for various consultants [25].

Media Response

Although the FDA response to the HRG petition was clear, the media response to the petition and its subsequent denial ranged from neutral to negative about the safety of piroxicam. Some news resports were objective and well balanced, but others were totally misleading. A Fort Lauderdale, Florida, broadcasting station inaccurately reported that piroxicam users were "completely safe." Another station took the position that the FDA had "refused to act" on the allegations that piroxicam was not safe, based on "inconclusive evidence," implying that there was still a question about piroxicam's relative safety, and that the FDA was irresponsible in taking no action. In New York, a CBS affiliate – watched by millions of viewers – reported that the government had not taken action against piroxicam and then reported all of the HRG allegations. This type of misinformation can do damage to a pharmaceutical company and is not in the best interest of the general public.

Piroxicam Sales

Not surprisingly, piroxicam prescribing decreased after the petition was filed in January 1986 and continued to decline even after the denial of the petition. Although sales eventually began to recover, Pfizer's promotion of the drug as well as physician and patient perception of the drug's safety were affected.

Sales Promotion

After the HRG petition raised questions about the relative safety of piroxicam, the same, unadjusted spontaneous report tables began to emerge in the competitive advertisements. The result was that piroxicam promotion had to take a defensive posture, basing subsequent advertising on the tenets of pharmacoepidemiology. Unfortunately the complexity of the issues of pharmacoepidemiology does not lend itself well to a drug detail situation.

Patient Perception

The patient population was also affected by the petition and related media attention. About one-third of patients surveyed were aware of the issues surrounding the petition. Approximately one-third of those patients who were aware subsequently stopped or changed medication because of the bad publicity [26]. Even drugs of the same class are not necessarily interchangeable on a patient-by-patient basis; an individual may not be as well treated if switched to another drug in the same therapeutic class. Such switching may increase the likelihood of a loss of efficacy or safety [27]. Similarly, physician prescription of piroxicam was also affected. Roughly 25% of physicians surveyed had at least one patient who asked to discontinue piroxicam because of publicity. Although there are good reasons for the patient to be involved in the choice of his or her medication, it is not sound medical practice for such decisions to be based on inaccurate publicity.

Conclusions

The existence of epidemiologic resources played a critical role in the defense of piroxicam against the scientifically unfounded attack. Had resources not been in place, the rapid assessment of piroxicam's relative safety could not have been carried out. Therefore, it is in the best interests of the pharmaceutical industry to continue to support the existing resources and to develop new ones that will be available and accessible to both industry and nonindustry investigators. The development of such resources is a gradual and lengthy process and industry support should come well *before* the need arises to evaluate a safety issue.

An equally important point is that scientifically valid pharmacoepidemiology plays a major role in furthering good public health practices [27]. This, in turn, serves industry since good public health may also be good for business. Conversely, poorly conducted pharmacoepidemiology based on unscientific methods may adversely affect public health considerations as well as the drug industry [27].

Finally, it is in industry's best interests to support training programs for epidemiologists specializing in drug safety. In this way, industry guarantees that it will have sufficient epidemiologic manpower in the future. Along with this support is the need to increase the awareness and understanding of the value of pharmacoepidemiology by industry, regulatory agencies, the public, and the media [27]. Industry must do its part to help this goal be realized.

References

1. Food and Drug Administration. Center for Drugs and Biologics (1984) Minutes of the Arthritis Advisory Committee meeting, Bethesda, Maryland, October 25–26
2. Food and Drug Administration. Center for Drugs and Biologics (1985) Minutes of the Arthritis Advisory Committee meeting, Bethesda, Maryland, April 29–30
3. Ferriman A (1985) "Arthritis Drug Alert After 77 Patients Die", The Observer, December 22
4. Letter to Secretary Bowen of the Department of Health and Human Services (1986) from Sidney Wolfe, Director, Health Research Group, January 8.
5. Transcript of Proceedings, United States of America before the Food and Drug Administration, In the Matter of: Piroxicam (1986) Docket Number 86P–0023, Bethesda, Maryland, February 28
6. Letter to Sidney M. Wolfe, Director, Health Research Group (1986) from Secretary Bowen of the Department of Health and Human Services, July 7
7. Pfizer Inc. (1986) Submission on the Petition of Public Citizen Health Research Group regarding Feldene (piroxicam), Food and Drug Administration, Docket Number 86P–0023, March 17
8. Food and Drug Administration, Center for Drugs and Biologics (1986) Recommendation in Piroxicam Imminent Hazard Proceeding, May 14
9. Memorandum to Secretary of Health and Human Services Otis Bowen (1986) from Frank E. Young, Commissioner, Food and Drug Administration, May 27
10. Sachs RM, Bortnichak EA (1986) An evaluation of spontaneous adverse drug reaction monitoring systems. Am J Med 81 (suppl 5B): 49–55
11. Weber JCP (1984) Epidemiology of adverse reactions to nonsteroidal anti-inflammatory drugs. In: Rainsford KD, Velo EP (eds) Advances in Inflammation Research Vol. 6. New York: Raven Press, pages 1–7
12. FDA (1986) personal communication
13. Meisel AD (1986) Clinical benefits and comparative safety of piroxicam: analysis of worldwide clinical trials data. Am J Med 81 (suppl 5B): 15–21
14. Bortnichak EA, Sachs RM (1986) Piroxicam in recent epidemiologic studies. Am J Med 81 (suppl 5B) 44–48
15. Stipp D (1988) "Scientists use medical-record data bases to detect adverse side-effects of drugs", The Wall Street Journal, March 24, p 33
16. Beard K, Walker AM, Perera DR, Jick H (1987) Nonsteroidal anti-inflammatory drugs and hospitalization for gastroesophageal bleeding in the elderly. Arch Intern Med 147: 1621–1623
17. Carson JL, Ștrom BL, Soper KA et al. (1987) The association of nonsteroidal anti-inflammatory drugs with upper gastrointestinal tract bleeding. Arch Intern Med 147: 85–88
18. Ray WA (1986) Tennessee Medicaid Database Study at Vanderbilt University. Correspondence (February 25)
19. Rawson NSB, Inman WHW (1986) Prescription-event monitoring: recent experience with 5 NSAIDs. Med Tox 1 (suppl 1): 79–82
20. Levy M, Miller DR, Kaufman DW, et al. (1988) Major upper gastrointestinal tract bleeding: relation to the use of aspirin and other nonnarcotic analgesics. Arch Intern Med 148: 281–285
21. Sommerville KW, Falkner G, Langman M (1986) Non-steroidal anti-inflammatory drugs and bleeding peptic ulcer. Lancet I: 462–464
22. Haglund U, Frost L, Wiholm BE: An evaluation of anti-inflammatory and analgesic drug intake among patients with acute gastrointestinal bleeding (abstr)

23. Giercksky KE, Revhaug A, Warloe T, et al. (1986) Can the incidence of gastrointestinal hemorrhage caused by drugs be reduced? Tidsskr Nor Laegeforen 106: 662–666
24. O'Brien JD, Burnham WR (1985) Bleeding from peptic ulcers and use of non-steroidal anti-inflammatory drugs in the Romford area. Br Med J 291: 1609–1610
25. The Pink Sheet (1987) In Brief: "The FDA's imbroglio", March 2
26. Data on file, Pfizer, Inc., New York
27. Sachs RM, Dieck GS (1987) Industry perspectives and the contributions of pharmacoepidemiology to public health. In: Edlavitch S (ed) Pharmacoepidemiology, Proceedings of the Third International Conference on Pharmacoepidemiology, Minneapolis (in press)

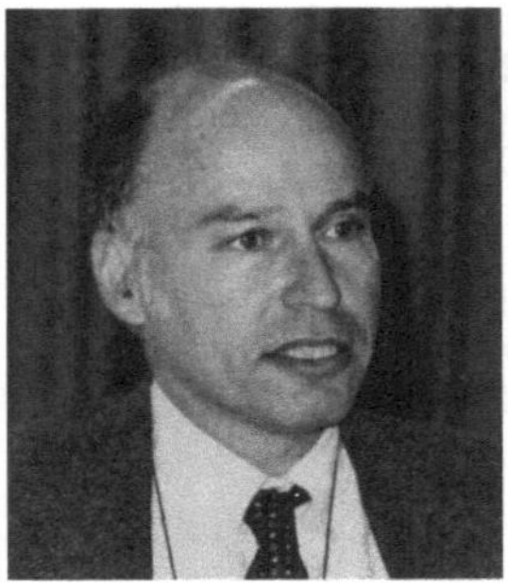

11. Risk Perception of Prescription Drugs: Report on a Survey in Sweden

P. Slovic, N. N. Kraus, H. Lappe, H. Letzel, and T. Malmfors

Introduction

RAD-AR, standing for risk assessment of drugs – analysis and response, is a program designed to improve the analysis and management of drug risks. Within the context of the RAD-AR program, risk perception has been designated as a priority research area. Knowledge of perception has been demonstrated to be vitally important in helping individuals and societies manage risks more effectively [4, 7]. In medicine, perceptions of drug risks are likely to influence patients' treatment choices, their compliance with treatment regimes, their views on the acceptability of adverse reactions, and their attitudes toward government regulation of drugs [9]. Understanding perceptions is a prerequisite for designing better communication materials for patients and the public. Yet most work in this area has focused on perceptions of risk from nuclear power, industrial chemicals, and other nonmedical hazards. Few, if any, studies have examined perceptions of pharmaceutical risks. The RAD-AR program is attempting to remedy this deficiency by means of a series of surveys designed to do the following:

1. Describe precisely and quantitatively the public's perceptions of risk and benefit from the use of various kinds of prescription drugs.
2. Place perceptions of prescription drugs within a broader context of risk perceptions regarding many other activities (e.g., driving, smoking) and technologies (e.g., air travel, pesticides), including other medical technologies (X rays, surgery).
3. Allow comparisons to be made across populations from different nations and, within national samples, across important personal and demographic characteristics (e.g., health status, age).
4. Provide baseline data that will allow the impact of new drug problems and controversies to be monitored and allow trends in relevant attitudes and perceptions to be followed over time.
5. Contribute to basic knowledge and understanding of the influence of public perceptions on the sociopolitical environment in which pharmaceutical companies operate.

This paper reports the results of the first survey in this series, which examined the attitudes and perceptions of a representative sample of the adult population of Sweden during March 1988.

Design and Administration of the Survey

Part I: General Attitudinal and Demographic Questionnaire

The survey had two separate components. Part I employed the traditional survey format in which respondents are asked to indicate their attitudes, perceptions, and opinions in response to specific questions. In addition, part I included a nontraditional task in which respondents were asked to read the words "prescription drugs" which were printed six times on a card. Each time they read these words, they were instructed to write down the first association that came to their minds. This technique, called the "method of continued associations", has been shown by Szalay and Deese [8] to be a sensitive indicator of the imagery and meaning associated with people's mental representations for a wide variety of concepts.

In addition to the imagery task, other questions in part I asked about the following:

- Perceptions of risk today as compared to risks in the past.
- Perceived frequency of side effects.
- The adequacy of performance by government regulators, drug manufacturers, doctors, and pharmacists in ensuring drug safety and efficacy.
- The respondent's personal experiences with drug side effects.
- Perceived causes of side effects.
- Opinions in response to a vignette describing a drug controversy.

Part I concluded with a series of demographic questions pertaining to the patient's age, sex, health status, cigarette smoking, occupation, income, marital status, medicine usage, health consciousness, attitude towards risk taking, attitude towards fate, and attitude toward using medicines.

Part II: Psychometric Questionnaire

During the past decade, standard questionnaires such as that used in part I above have been supplemented by more quantitative studies in what has come to be known as the psychometric paradigm for studying risk perception [6, 7]. Within this paradigm people are asked to make quantitative judgments about the riskiness of various hazards. Perceptions of risk are then related statistically to quantitative judgments of other properties of the hazards being studied, such as the degree to which the risks are known to those exposed to them or the seriousness of harm in the event of an accident or mishap.

In the present survey, quantitative judgments were made for each of the 29 items shown in Table 11.1. These items included 15 pharmaceutical products (eg., vaccines, antibiotics, etc.), five medical devices or procedures (e. g., X rays, heart surgery), and nine nonmedical items (e. g., automobiles, nuclear power) included to provide a broad context against which to compare and contrast the medical and pharmaceutical items. The pharmaceutical items were carefully selected according to several criteria, including importance, familiarity to the general public, and diversity. Although we wanted to include more than 15 pharmaceutical items, doing so would have made the survey too time consuming.

Table 11.1. Hazard items studied in Part II

1. Pharmaceutical items	
Vaccines	Anticancer drugs
Laxatives	Aspirin
Antibiotic drugs	Herbal medicines
Birth control pills	Vitamin pills
Insulin	Antiarthritics
Sleeping pills	Biotechnology drugs
Antihypertensives	Drugs against AIDS
Antidepressants	
2. Medical procedures, tests, and devices	
Medical X rays	Acupuncture
IUDs	Appendectomy
Heart surgery	
3. Nonmedical hazards	
Automobiles	Artificial sweeteners
Travel by airplane	Food additives
Nuclear power plants	Alcoholic beverages
Pesticides	Cigarette smoking
Household cleansers	

Each of the 29 items was rated by each respondent on seven characteristics of risk, similar to those found to be important in prior studies of perceived risk [7]. In addition to rating the perceived risk and perceived benefit for each item, respondents rated the extent to which the risks are known to those exposed to them, the likelihood that people exposed to the risk would experience any degree of personal harm, the extent to which the risk associated with each item was new or old, the seriousness of harmful effects in the event of an accident or mishap, and the degree to which a mishap would serve as a warning sign indicating that the risk from this item might be greater than was thought before the problem occurred. The full set of rating scales for these seven characteristics is shown in Table 11.2. All 29 hazard items were rated on one scale before the next scale was considered. Before starting this task, respondents were asked to examine a glossary which defined each term (e.g., insulin – a drug used to treat diabetes).

A primary contribution of previous risk-perception research has been to show that qualities of risk such as those surveyed in the present study determine important societal responses to hazards. For example, acceptability of risk usually relates positively to perceived benefit and negatively to perceived risk. Hazards posing risks that are judged to be new, not well known, and serious, such as chemical manufacturing or nuclear power, also tend to be judged most in need of strict governmental regulation. And when these "worrisome" technologies experience an accident, the mishap is likely to be interpreted as a "warning signal" (scale 7) indicating that the responsible company, and perhaps also the industry, is not managing the risks properly [7]. Such signals may trigger strong societal reactions or "ripple effects" (public opposition, liability suits, stricter government regulation, product withdrawals) that can inflict massive costs on a company or industry [3]. A dramatic example of

Table 11.2. Scales on which the 29 items were rated

Risk to those exposed
To what extent would you say that people (for instance you or someone you know) who are exposed to this item are at risk of experiencing personal harm from it? (1 = they are not at risk; 7 = they are very much at risk)

Benefits
In general, how beneficial do you consider this item to be for society as a whole? (1 = not at all beneficial; 7 = very beneficial)

Likelihood of harm
How likely would you say it is that people who are exposed to this item actually *will experience* any type of personal harm, mild or serious? (1 = very unlikely to experience harm; 7 = very likely to experience harm)

Seriousness of harm
If an accident or unfortunate event involving this item occurred, to what extent are the harmful effects to a person likely to be mild, or serious? (1 = very mild harm; 7 = very serious harm)

Knowledge of those exposed
To what extent would you say that the risks associated with this item are known precisely to people who are exposed to those risks? (1 = risk level known; 7 = risk level not known)

Old or new risk
To what extent is this item a new risk, or an old one that has been around for a long time? (1 = very old; 7 = very new)

Warning sign
If you read in the newspaper about an accident or an illness involving this item, in which people were seriously harmed, to what degree would this mishap serve as a warning sign, indicating that the *risk of this item might be greater* than was thought before the problem occurred? (1 = not a warning sign; 7 = very strong warning sign)

ripple effects followed the accident at the Three Mile Island nuclear reactor. This mishap was estimated to have cost tens (perhaps hundreds) of billions of dollars as a result of reduced output from nuclear reactors worldwide, costs of using more expensive alternative fuels, stricter regulation of the industry, etc. [1, 2]. The Ford Pinto, the gas tank of which was prone to explode in a collision, is an obvious example of an extremely serious and costly defect for the automobile industry, both in terms of the monetary costs of litigation and intangible losses of good will and public regard for the manufacturer.

The scales included in this survey were selected with the intent of assessing the potential for costly ripple effects in the event of mishaps involving specific pharmaceutical products. In addition, the quantitative judgments of risk and benefit (along with the imagery data from Part I) can serve as sensitive baseline data against which to monitor changes in perceptions over time.

Administration of the Survey

A representative sample of the Swedish adult population between the ages of 16 and 74 was interviewed in their own homes by personnel from SIFO, a leading survey and market research firm in Sweden. The interviews took place from February 24 through March 19, 1988. Due to the lengthy psychometric scaling task (Part II), some persons needed as much as 90 min to complete the interview. Nevertheless, from 1234 persons contacted, 961 completed interviews were obtained, for a completion rate of 78%.

Results of Part I

Characteristics of the Sample

The sample was about equally split between women (50.4%) and men (49.6%). About 28% of the respondents resided in Stockholm or Gothenberg; 17% resided in small villages (less than 3000 inhabitants) or rural areas; the remaining 55% came from towns and cities of intermediate size. Most of the respondents were between the ages of 16 and 39 (47.3%), 34.8% were between the ages of 40 and 59, and 17.9% were between 60 and 74 years of age.

The majority of respondents rated their health as either excellent (34.6%) or very good (28.4%); 30.2% rated their health as fair and 6.6% as poor. When asked if they had a chronic illness or condition, 12.7% answered yes.

Some 20.9% of the sample said that they saw their doctor regularly; 27.0% had bought a nonprescription medicine within the previous 4 months; 62.5% said they had benefited significantly during the past 5 years from taking a prescription drug. As expected, a much higher percentage of the patients who described themselves as chronically ill had received a prescription drug during the past 4 months (68%) than those who had no chronic illness (37%).

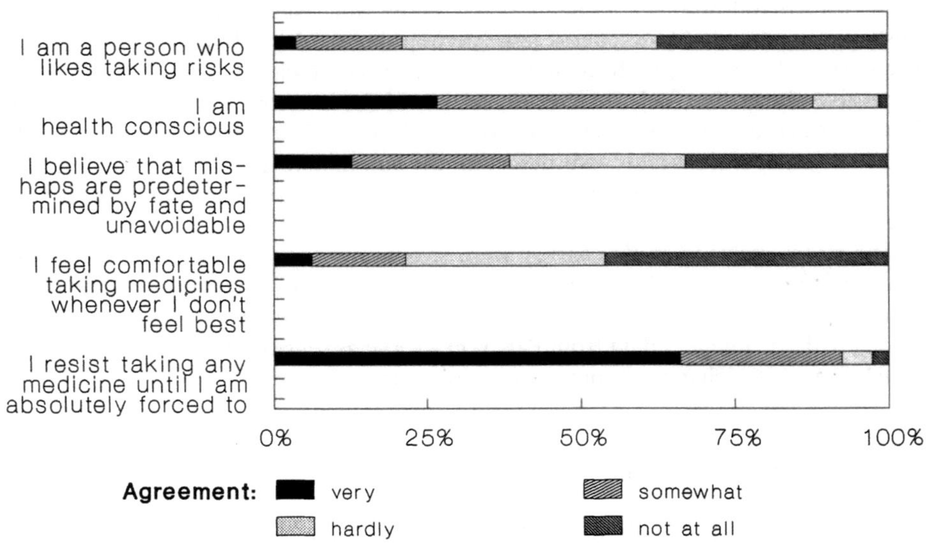

Fig. 11.1. Attitudes toward health, risk, fate, and medicines

Respondents were asked to indicate the degree to which various statements about risk taking, health consciousness, fatalism, and medicine taking described them personally. The results, shown in Fig. 11.1 indicate that most of these individuals characterized themselves as not liking to take risks, being health conscious, not feeling comfortable about taking medicines, and resisting the use of medicine until they are absolutely forced to do so (92.2% said they were very or somewhat well characterized by this last statement). There was more divergence of views regarding fate. About 38% said they believed most mishaps in life are predetermined by fate and are unavoidable; 61% said that such beliefs did not describe their personal view.

Images of Prescription Drugs

More than 3000 associations were produced in response to the stimulus concept "prescription drugs." The major types of associations are listed in Table 11.3 in order

Table 11.3. Associations with "prescription drugs"

Rank	Association	Count
1	All names of drugs (i.e., valium, etc.)	549
2	All states of illness	465
3	Types of drugs, e.g., antibiotics, vitamins	412
4	"Medicine," i.e., liquid form, syrup	299
5	Pills	261
6	Hospital	258
7	Doctor	222
8	Helpful	188
9	Industry, research, company	161
10	Side effects	136
11	Pharmacy	132
12	Natural, herbal medicine	92
13	Abuse	81
14	Dangerous	78
15	Recovery, healing	60
16	Addiction, dependence	45
17	Prescriptions	42
18	Price, money, cost	33
19	Overdose, overconsumption	26
20	Hypodermic needle	24
21	Bottles, jars, boxes	23
22	Warning	22
23	Profit	21
24	Paraphernalia (general)	18
25	Allergy, reactions	10
26	Preservatives	9
27	Death	7
28	Effective	7
29	Reliable, guaranteed	4

of their frequency. Names of drugs headed the list, followed closely by states and names of illnesses and types of drugs. Strong positive images (helpful, recovery, healing, effective, reliable) accounted for 259 responses. Strong negative imagery was somewhat more frequent and took two general forms: one form had to do with side effects, dangerousness, warning, allergic and other reactions, and death (total frequency of this form, 253); the other had to do with abuse, addiction, dependency, overdose, and overconsumption (total frequency, 152). Natural and herbal medicines were mentioned 92 times. Cost was mentioned rather infrequently.

Surveys of limited samples of young adults in the United States have shown that associations with the word "chemicals" are dominated by negative imagery (death, toxic, dangerous). The Swedish data show that responses to one class of chemicals, prescription drugs, are much more neutral and positive. Overall, the data in Table 11.3 seem to provide a useful baseline against which to compare responses over time in Sweden and responses from other nations.

Present and Past Risk

Respondents were asked to indicate whether they believed that there is more risk, less risk, or about the same risk today than there was 20 years ago for each of several types of hazard. The results, shown in Fig. 11.2, indicate that the risks from chemicals were

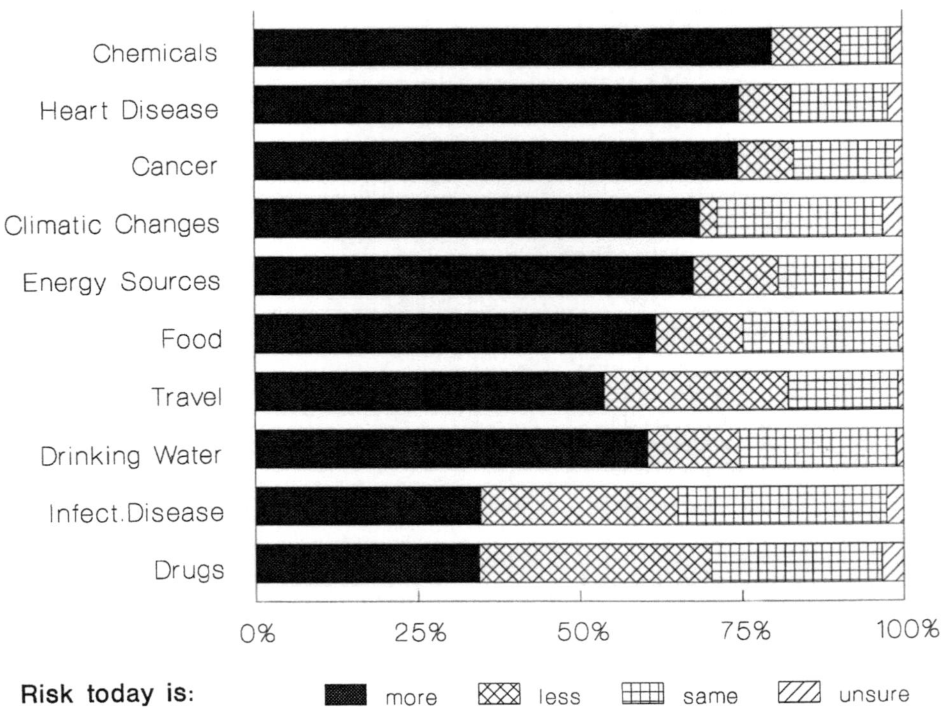

Fig. 11.2. Risk today versus 20 years ago

perceived to be greater today by 80% of the respondents. Other percentages for the "more risk" response were heart disease (75%), cancer (74%), climate changes (69%), energy sources (67%), food (62%), quality of drinking water (60%), methods of travel (54%), infectious diseases excluding AIDS (35%), and prescription drugs (34%). Looking at the other side of the coin, the proportion of responses in the "less risk today" category was highest for prescription drugs (35.8%) and infectious diseases (30.4%) and lowest for climate changes (2.7%).

We thus see a strong differentiation in the perceived trend in risk between prescription drugs and other chemicals as well as between drugs and other technologies. Although about one-third of the Swedish sample believes that drug risks have increased, this is far smaller than the percentage perceiving increased risk from the other hazards, with the exception of infectious disease, which may be seen as closely linked to drug efficacy.

Drug Efficacy and Side Effects

Several questions asked about drug efficacy and the frequency, severity, and causes of side effects. When asked to rate the job that various health-care agents were doing to make sure that prescription drugs are safe and effective, pharmacists received the highest marks (70% excellent or good), followed at quite a distance by doctors (56%), government regulatory agencies (50%), and drug manufacturers (40%), as shown in Fig. 11.3. The small percentage of excellent ratings for every group suggests that, in the public mind, there is room for improvement in this matter.

When asked how often patients taking prescription drugs experience *serious* side effects, 23.5% replied always, very often, or often. When asked whether they personally had suffered a side effect from taking a prescription drug during the past 5 years,

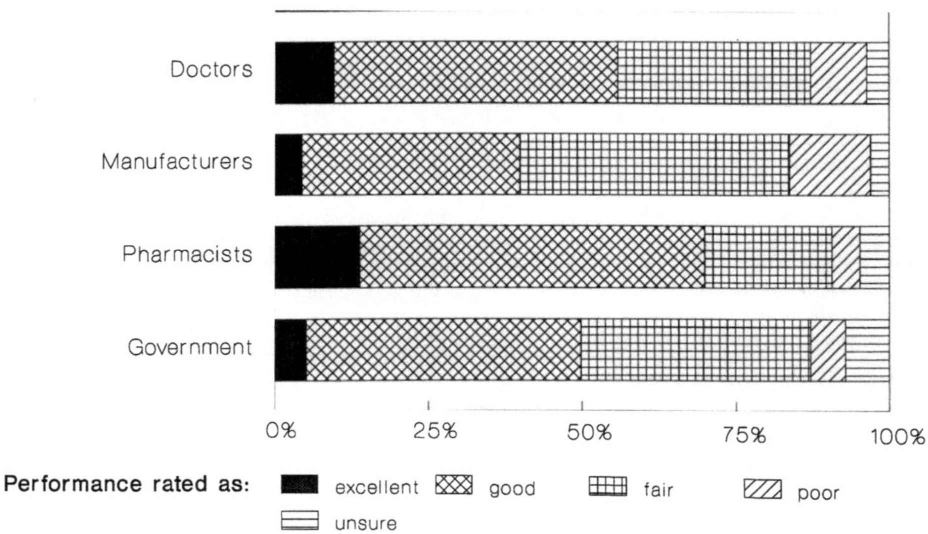

Fig. 11.3. Ensuring safety and efficacy: confidence in selected health care groups

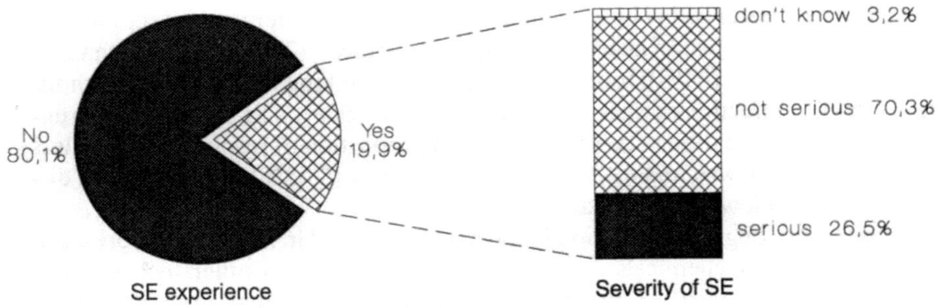

Fig. 11.4. Side effect (*SE*) experience within the past 5 years

19.9% replied yes (see Fig. 11.4); of these, 26.5% considered the side effect serious. Multiplying these two proportions indicates that only 5.3% of the total sample claimed to have suffered a serious side effect, a proportion far smaller than that attributed to other patients who take prescription drugs.

Respondents were also asked to indicate their opinions about the main cause of a drug side effect. Their spontaneous responses, shown in Table 11.4, named patient sensitivity, improper drug prescription or wrong diagnosis, and noncompliance as the major causes. Following this question was a structured question that asked people to indicate how frequently each of eight specified factors is the cause of a side effect. The results, shown in Fig. 11.5, indicate that patient sensitivity was again singled out as one of the most frequent causal factors (44.5% rated it always, very often, or often a cause). Improper monitoring of the patient by the doctor was rated similarly frequent (45% always, very often, or often). Slightly less frequent attributions of causality were assigned to failure to adequately inform the patient (41%), lack of patient compliance (38%), and inadequate health and safety testing by the manufacturer (38%). Again pharmacist's mistakes were seen as the least likely causes (2%).

Table 11.4. Reasons for side effects: spontaneous mentions

Reason	Frequency
Patient allergic	33.2%
Wrong drug, diagnosis	27.9%
Noncompliance	13.5%
Drug interaction	8.7%
New, untried drug	8.4%
Insufficient control	6.0%
Poor information	5.5%
No answer	5.3%

Basis, 1942 spontaneous mentions

A Drug Crisis Scenario

The following hypothetical scenario was posed to each respondent, indicating a possible link between a drug and some fatalities among its users.

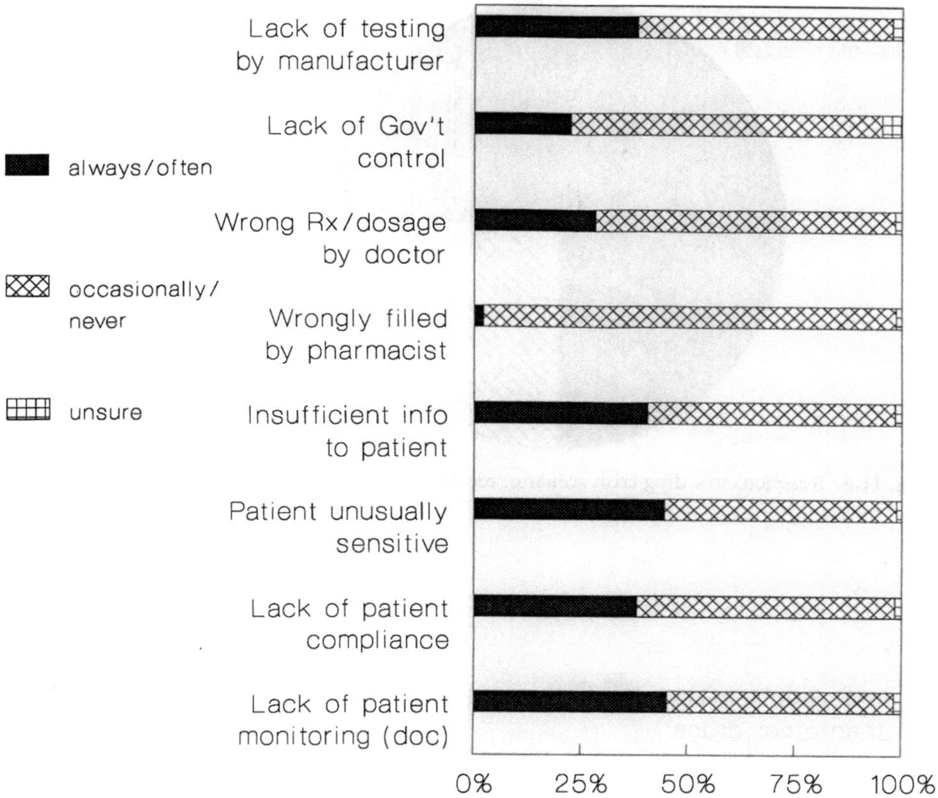

Fig. 11.5. Reasons for side effects: prompted responses

"Imagine that a new prescription drug becomes available in this country for treating a serious disease. Other drugs are also available for treating this disease. A study reveals that some people may have died from taking this drug. What do you think the government should do in this case?
- Leave the drug on the market.
- Take the drug off the market.
- Leave the drug on the market, but warn doctors and patients.
- Not sure."

As Fig. 11.6 indicates, 75% of respondents wanted the government to take the drug off the market; 1.8% wanted the drug left on the market, and another 21.8% wanted it left on the market with a warning.

Those who wanted the drug removed from the market or were not sure (76.7% of the total sample) were asked to reconsider their answers, taking into account each of six possible extenuating circumstances. The results, shown in Fig. 11.7, indicate that there is no circumstance that, by itself, would convince more than 16% of these people to leave the drug on the market. However, in combination with information warning

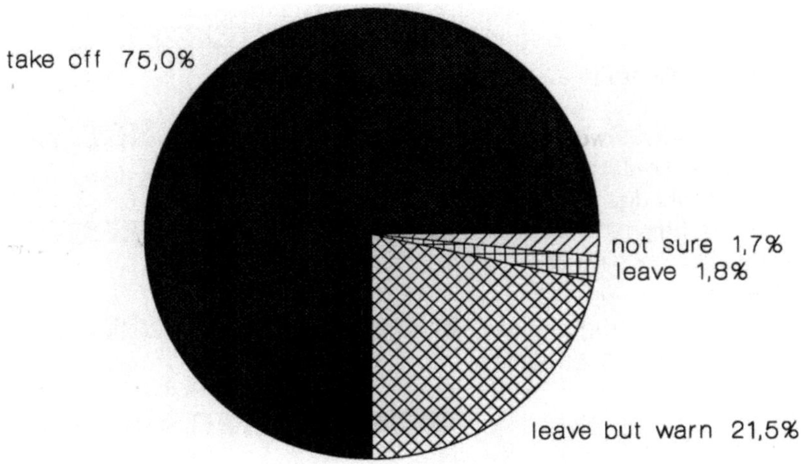

Fig. 11.6. Reactions to a drug crisis scenario: recommended government action

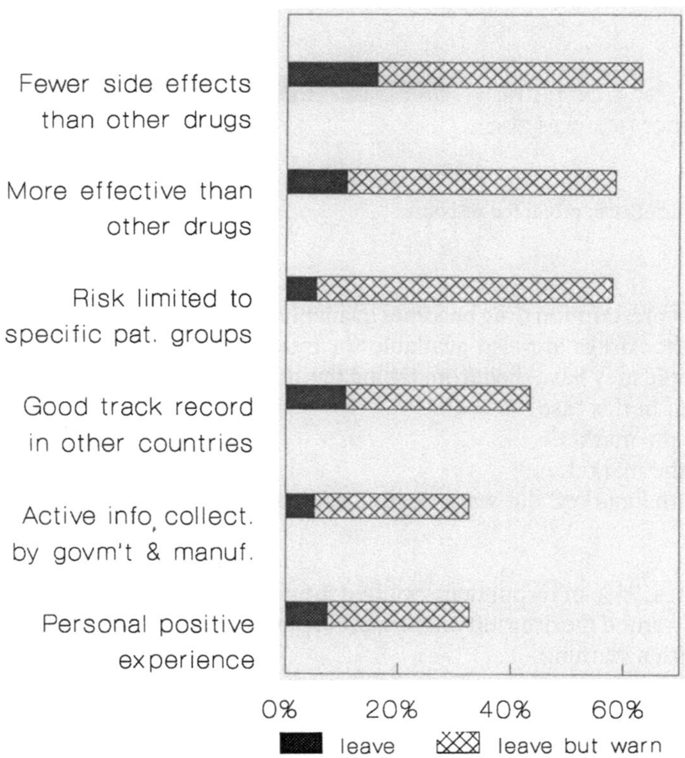

Fig. 11.7. Reactions to a drug crisis scenario: modification of opinion in view of additional evidence. Basis: those wanting the drug removed from the market or were not sure (see Fig. 11.6)

doctors and patients about the possible problem, these circumstances led to considerable change in opinions. Knowledge that the risk affected only certain types of patients convinced 5.4% of these respondents to leave the drug on the market and another 52.6% to leave it on the market with a warning. Changes such as this also occurred when respondents were told that the drug is more effective than other, similar drugs, or that the drug has fewer side effects for most patients than other, similar drugs. Being told that the drug has been used safely and effectively for many years in another country produced somewhat less change in opinions. The two circumstances that produced the least opinion change were the fact that the government and manufacturer are actively gathering more information about the problem and the fact that the respondent had taken the drug for many months and was very satisfied with it.

Analysis of sample subgroups indicated that those who were not comfortable taking medicines, those who had suffered side effects during the past 5 years, those who do not like taking risks, and those in the younger age groups were most likely to want the drug withdrawn from the market upon hearing of possible deaths from taking it. The age factor had the largest effect. About 76% of respondents aged 59 or younger

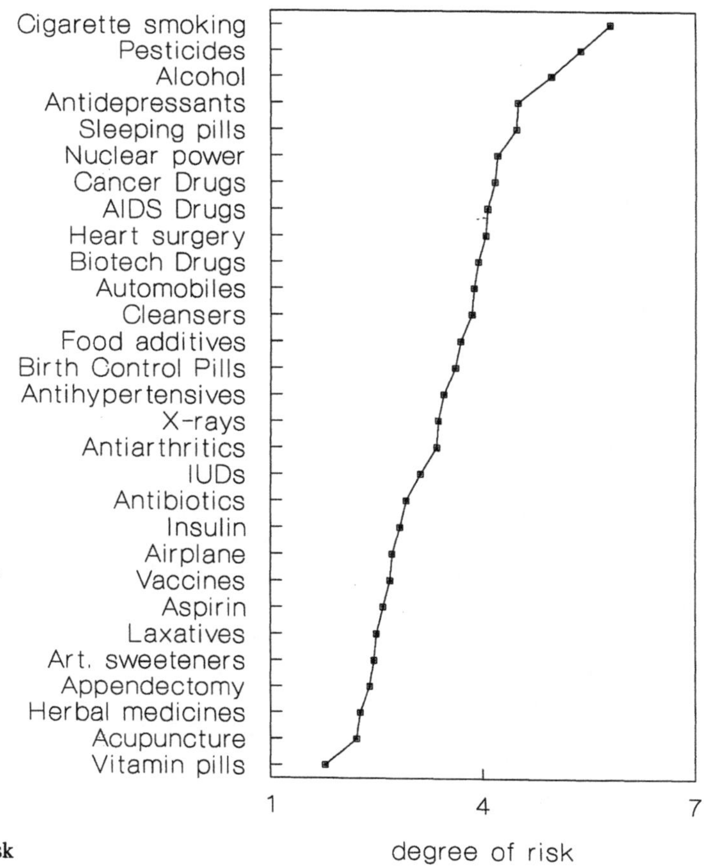

Fig. 11.8. Perceived risk

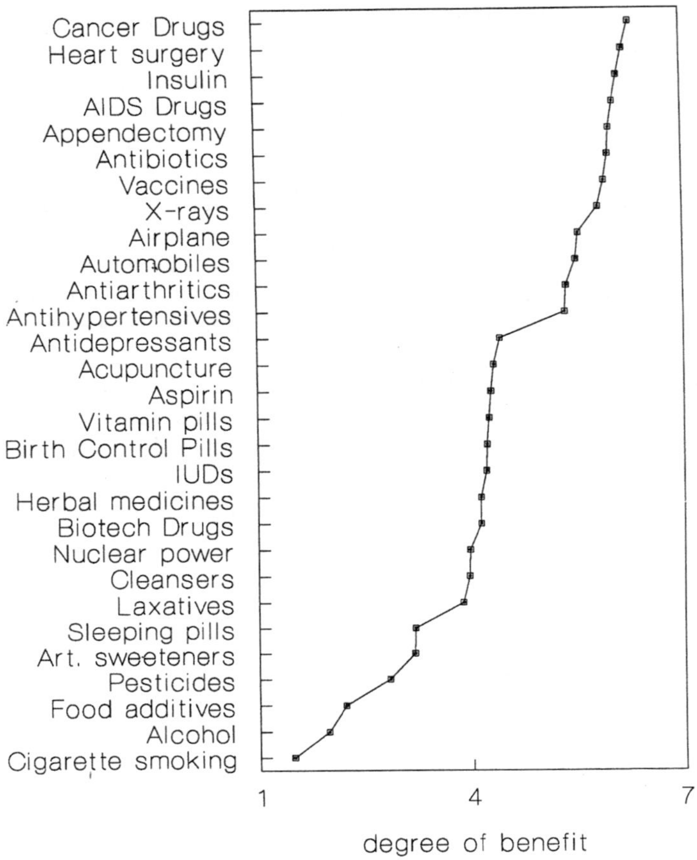

Fig. 11.9. Perceived benefit

wanted to have the drug withdrawn after hearing about the study report, while only 66% of persons in the 60–74 age bracket wanted it withdrawn. In the second part of the question, older people were much more tolerant about leaving the drug on the market while the government and manufacturer gathered more information about the problem. One exception to this tolerance occurred when the risk of death was said to affect only certain types of patients. In this case only 34.5% and 39.8%, respectively, of those in the 16–39 and 40–59 age ranges wanted the drug withdrawn, but 45.2% of those in the oldest age group wanted it withdrawn, perhaps fearing that older patients were the ones most at risk.

The greater tolerance for risk demonstrated by older persons on most of the scenario questions may be due to the fact that older people are more dependent upon medicines. This, in turn, suggests that a sample of patients might respond differently from our predominantly healthy sample to questions about drug withdrawals.

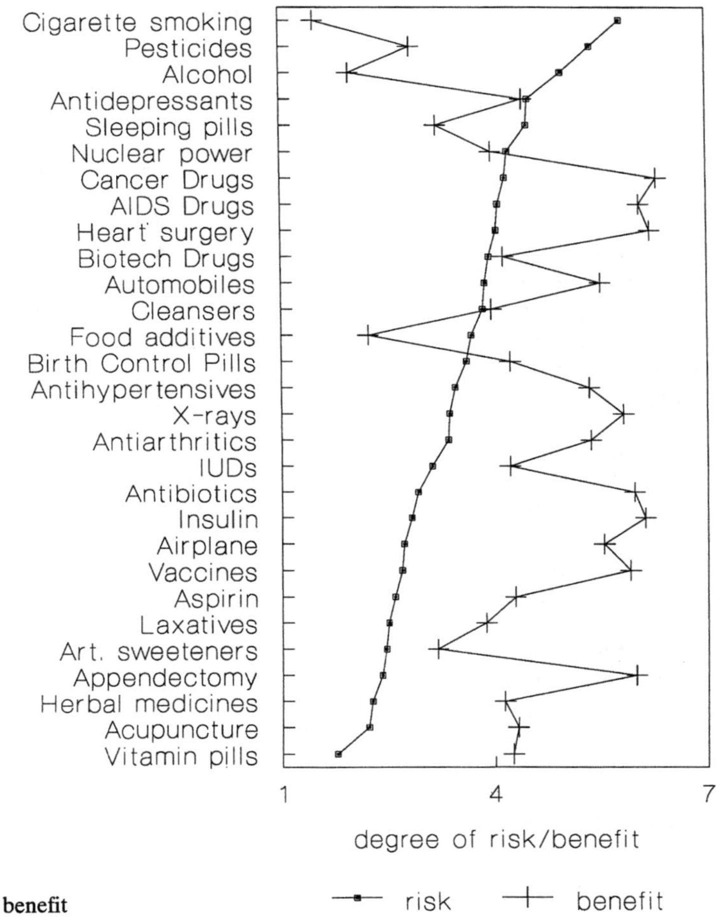

Fig. 11.10. Risk and benefit

Results of the Psychometric Questionnaire

Ratings of each hazard item were averaged across all 961 respondents for each scale. The mean ratings for perceived risk, ordered from high to low, are shown in Fig. 11.8. Three nondrug chemicals – cigarette smoking, pesticides, and alcohol – stand out as highest in perceived risk, followed by two drug items – antidepressants and sleeping pills – which, surprisingly, are judged more risky than nuclear power. Vitamin pills, acupuncture, and herbal medicines were judged lowest in risk.

Analysis of means for specific subgroups of respondents showed that women perceived far higher risk from nuclear power than did men (mean rating, 4.86 for women and 3.53 for men; $p < .001$). This is a common finding in studies of perceived risk. However, no other differences between men and women exceeded .4. Those who claimed to have experienced any sort of side effect from a prescription drug showed slightly higher mean perceptions of risk than those without side effect experi-

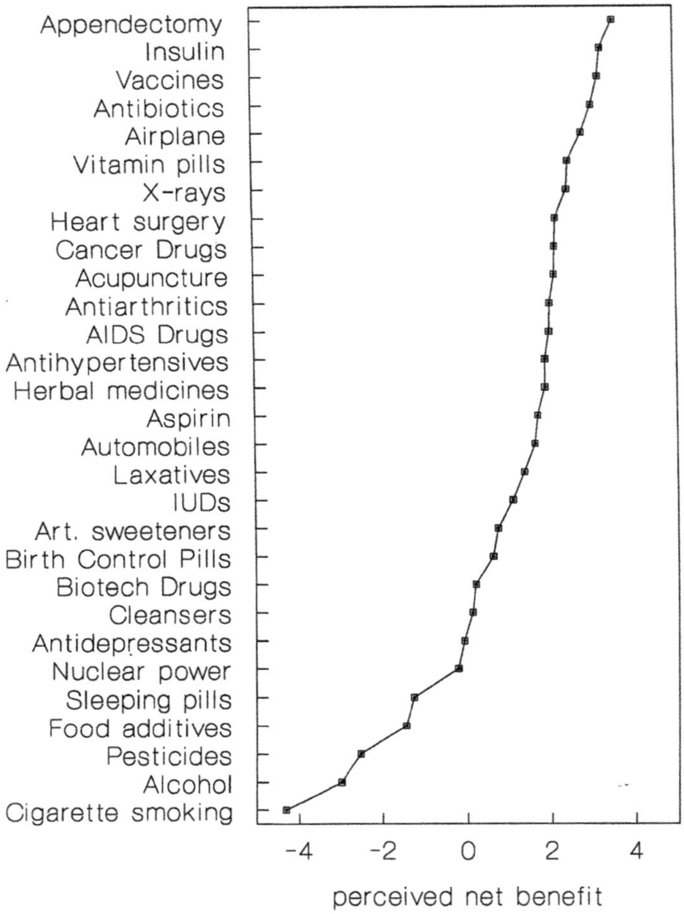

Fig. 11.11. Net benefit

ence (the largest mean difference was .57 for antibiotics; $p < .001$). Perceptions of risk seemed unaffected by having experienced significant benefits from taking drugs.

Mean ratings of perceived benefit are shown in Fig. 11.9. Unlike mean perceptions of risk, which exhibited a smooth, continuous decline from high to low values, benefits seem to fall into three categories. High benefits are associated with cancer drugs, heart surgery, insulin, AIDS drugs, appendectomy, antibiotics, vaccines, X rays, airplanes, automobiles, and drugs to treat arthritis and hypertension. Moderate benefits are attributed to 11 items ranging from antidepressants to laxatives. Very low benefits are perceived for cigarettes, alcohol, food additives, pesticides, artificial sweeteners, and sleeping pills. The perceived benefit of various drug items was only slightly higher for those claiming to have experienced significant benefits in the past 5 years than for those not claiming such beneficial experiences.

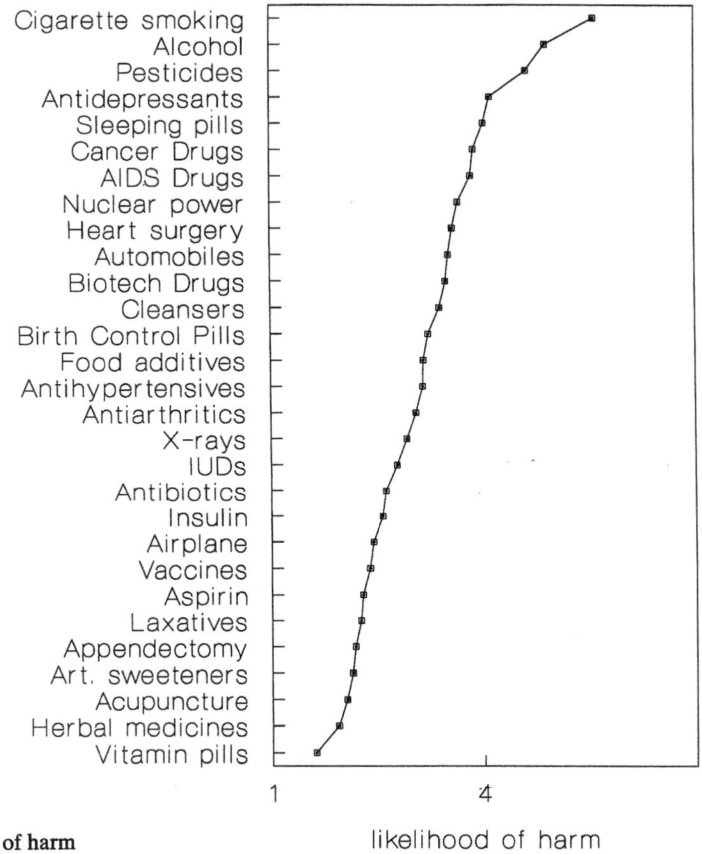

Fig. 11.12. Likelihood of harm

The risk and benefit means are superimposed in Fig. 11.10. It is obvious that perceived risks and benefits are not positively related (the correlation is actually − .23). Some items are of low risk and high benefit (e.g., appendectomy) and others the opposite (e.g., cigarettes). Assuming that the seven-point scales are commensurate, we can subtract the benefit mean from the risk mean for each item, producing the scale of mean net benefits shown in Fig. 11.11. According to this analysis, appendectomy, insulin, vaccines, and antibiotics are judged highest in net benefit. Vitamin pills are not far behind. Four nondrug chemicals – cigarettes, alcohol, pesticides, and food additives – show the most negative net benefits. Most drug items have positive net benefits, except for antidepressants and sleeping pills.

Subgroup analysis showed that the perceived net benefits for antidepressants, birth controll pills, sleeping pills, and antihypertensives were higher for those persons claiming to be comfortable taking medicines than for those who are not comfortable doing so. However, these two groups of people did not differ in their net benefit ratings for such high-benefit drugs as vaccines, antibiotics, and insulin. Older respon-

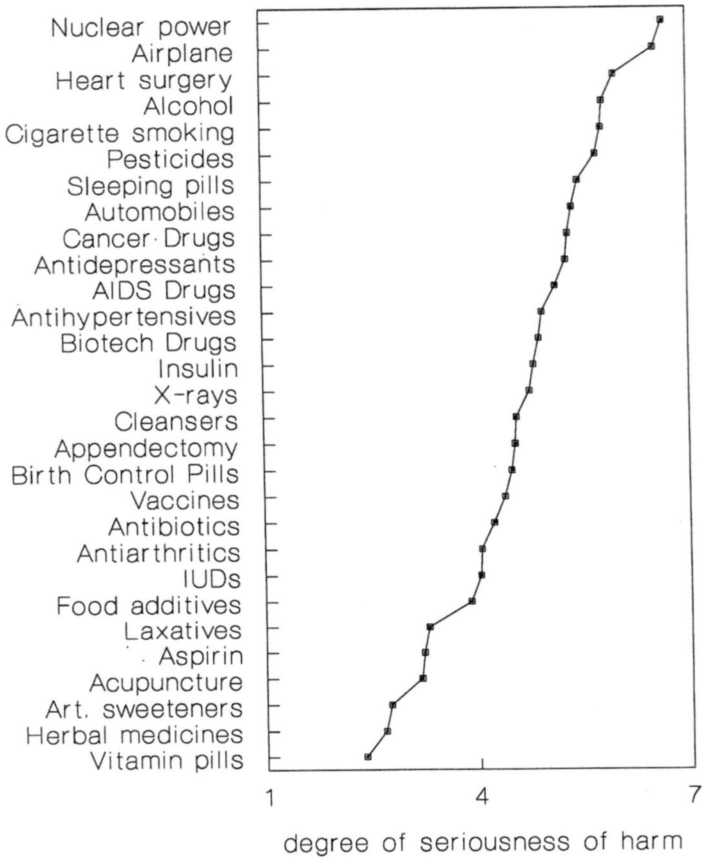

Fig. 11.13. Seriousness of harm

dents (ages 60–74) showed slightly higher net benefit ratings for antihypertensives, cancer drugs, antidepressants, and artificial sweeteners.

Figures 11.12–11.16 present the ordered means for the remaining five scales: likelihood of harm, seriousness of harm, knowledge of risk among those exposed to it, newness of the risk, and the strength of the warning signal that would be triggered by a mishap involving the hazard item. Likelihood of harm (Fig. 11.12) was almost perfectly correlated with perceived risk ($r = .996$). Seriousness ratings (Fig. 11.13) differed from likelihood ratings in that nuclear power, airplanes, and heart surgery moved to the highest ranks. Knowledge of risk (Fig. 11.14) took an intermediate position for all items – there was rather little variation from the least well known risks (biotechnology drugs, food additives) to the best known (airplanes, automobiles, and cigarettes). There was much greater variation on the new versus old scale (Fig. 11.15) ranging from AIDS and biotechnology drugs (newest risks) to cigarettes and alcohol (oldest). The warning sign scale also showed rather small variation around the midpoint (Fig. 11.16). Nuclear power and pesticides were highest on this scale, and automobiles and airplanes were lowest.

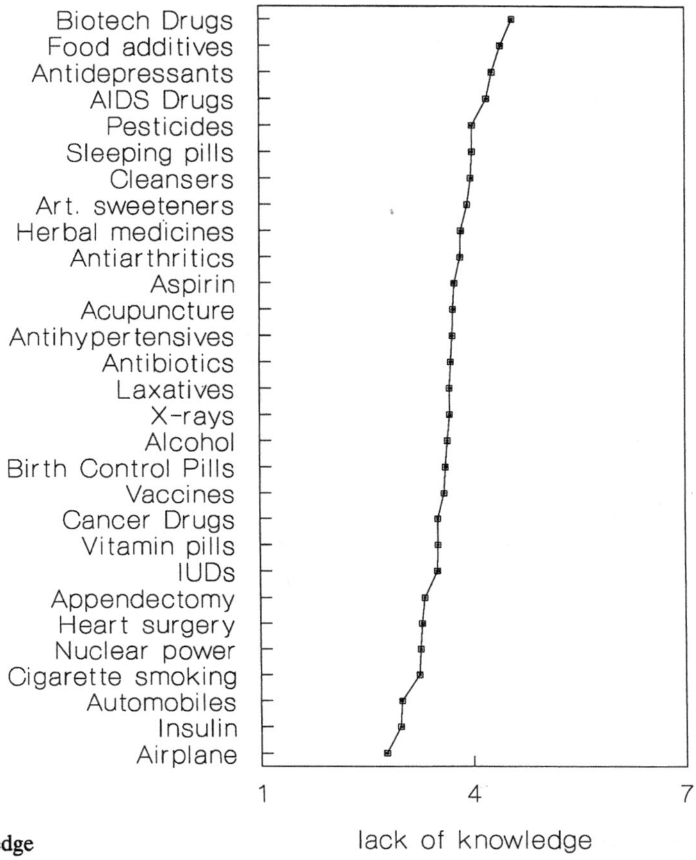

Fig. 11.14. Risk knowledge

Correlation coefficients were calculated between the means of each pair of scales, across the 29 items. These correlations were subjected to a principal components factor analysis which uncovered two dominant, uncorrelated factors accounting for 71% of the variance in the scales. Factor I, which we label "risk", consisted of three scales: perceived risk, the likelihood of harm, and the seriousness of harm, given a mishap. Factor II, which we call "warning", consisted of the scales pertaining to newness, knowledge, and warning sign. Factor scores were computed for each hazard item by weighting the mean ratings on each scale proportionally to the importance of that scale for the factor and summing over all scales. The weighted sum gives each item a score that is an amalgamation of its ratings on the scales that define each factor. The factor scores for each item are plotted in Fig. 11.17. As one moves from left to right in the factor space, the items are judged to have higher likelihood of causing harm, greater severity of harm in the event of a mishap, and, overall. greater perceived risk. As one goes from the bottom to the top of the space, the items are judged to have risks that are newer and less precisely known, and a mishap is judged as providing a stronger warning about the possibility that the risk is greater than was previously believed.

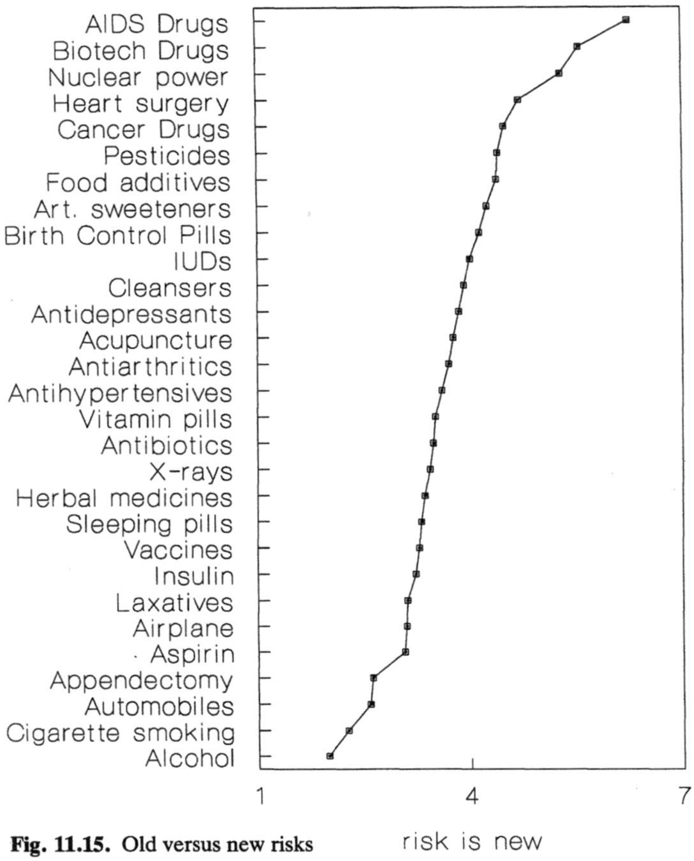

Fig. 11.15. Old versus new risks

As we would expect from the mean ratings shown in Fig. 11.14 (knowledge) and 11.16 (warning sign), most pharmaceutical products cluster together at an intermediate level on Factor II. However, there is great differentiation on the risk factor, with sleeping pills and antidepressant drugs seen as extremely high in risk. Nuclear power and pesticides are judged as new, unknown, and high-risk technologies and are located in the upper-right quadrant of the space, much as previous studies have shown. Drugs against AIDS and drugs made by means of biotechnology are seen as new and unknown risks, and relatively higher in perceived risk than most other pharmaceutical products.

Discussion

A prior survey of risk attitudes in Sweden, conducted by SIFO in January 1988, demonstrated extremely great public concern about the risks from chemicals. Some 81% of those interviewed agreed with the statement that "It can never be too

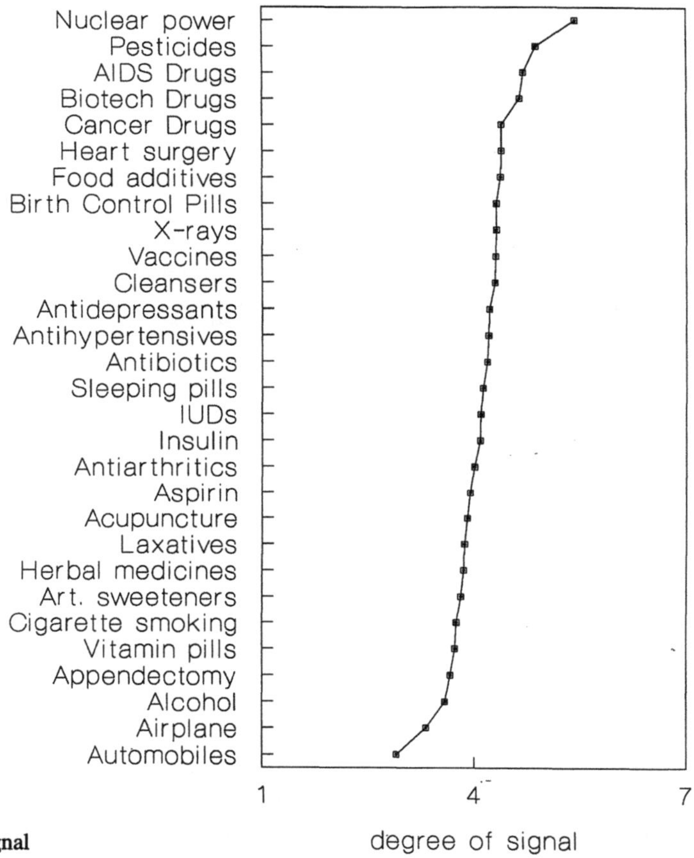

Fig. 11.16. Warning signal

expensive to reduce the risks from chemicals". An even stronger anti-chemical statement – "All use of chemicals must be risk free" – drew agreement from 75% of the respondents. Such concerns were exhibited in the present survey in which 80% of the respondents stated that risks from chemicals are greater today than they were 20 years ago. In addition, chemical items such as food additives and pesticides were rated extremely high in risk and low in benefit. Besides being greatly concerned about chemical risks, the Swedish respondents in the present survey characterized themselves as persons who disliked taking risks, and who resisted taking medicines unless forced to do so.

Given these attitudes, we could expect to find rather harsh views in Sweden about the risks from another class of chemicals – prescription drugs. For the most part, this was not the case. Prescription drugs, with the exception of sleeping pills and antidepressants, were perceived as rather high in benefit and low in risk. They appeared to be sharply differentiated from other chemicals and from illicit drugs. The concerns about sleeping pills and antidepressants perhaps can be traced to extensive media publicity during recent years regarding the risks of addiction and overdose from these and similar drugs.

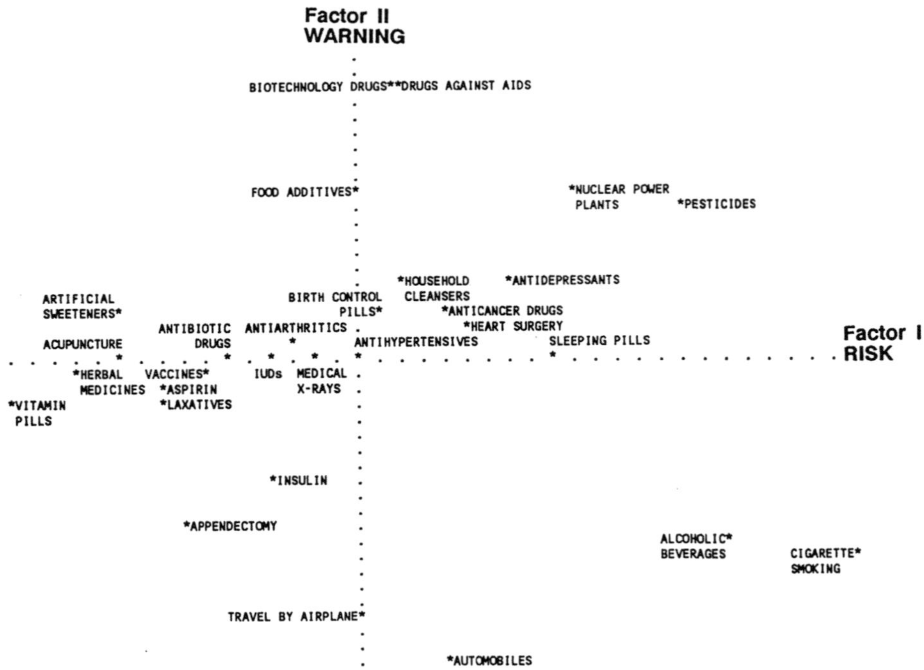

Fig. 11.17. Perceptual map of risk factors

Although mishaps involving prescription drugs were judged to produce only moderate warning signals, the scenario item from Part I of the survey showed the potential for a strong reaction to the report of a suspected but not proven link between a drug and some fatalities. At a hint of trouble, 75% of those surveyed wanted the drug removed from the market. However, one of the most intriguing findings in this study was the indication that evidence of safety and efficacy, in combination with warning information, could reverse a high proportion of these initial demands for withdrawal of the drug.

The strategy of marketing a drug to a carefully targeted patient population, coupled with thorough warnings about its risks, is currently being pursued by the Alza Corporation in their marketing of the IUD, Progestasert. The response to the scenario item in the present survey suggests that appropriate use of warnings may be an important general strategy for decreasing the vulnerability of prescription drugs. This suggestion should certainly be investigated in future studies.

The present study demonstrates the potential usefulness of survey research for describing and monitoring key attitudes and perceptions regarding drug risks. Replication of this type of study in other countries and with samples of patients rather than members of the general public should prove valuable.

Acknowledgments. This study was sponsored by Ciba-Geigy, Ltd. in Basel, Switzerland. Walter von Wartburg and Günter Lewandowski provided support and encouragement throughout all phases of the study. Many others made valuable contributions to the design, execution, and analysis of the study. We wish to give special thanks to David Taylor, Dana Miller, Merl Baker, Johan Werner, Stig Arne Ekedahl, George Wistrom, Ernst Bluemner, Elizabeth Moench, Nancy Mattison, Edward Bortnichak, Buddy Prettyman, Marvin Wetter, Dennis Burley, Bernie O'Brien, Gwen Parr, Rolf Dinkel, C.R.B. Joyce, D. Mac Gregor, Ursula Schmid, and Viveka Linde.

References

1. EPRI Journal (1980) Assessment: the impact and influence of TMI. Electric Power Research Institute, Palo Alto, California 5(5), 24–33
2. Evans N, Hope CW (1982) Costs of nuclear accidents: implications for reactor choice. Energy Policy 295–304
3. Kasperson RE, Renn O, Slovic P, Brown HS, Emel G, Goble R, Kasperson JX, Ratick S (1988) The social amplification of risk: a conceptual framework. Risk Analysis, 8, 177–187
4. The Royal Society (1983) Risk assessment: report of a Royal Society study group. London
5. Slovic P, Lichtenstein S, Fischhoff B (1984) Modeling the societal impact of fatal accidents. Management Science, 30: 464–474
6. Slovic P, Fischhoff B, Lichtenstein S (1985) Characterizing perceived risk. In Kates RW, Hohenemser C, Kasperson JX (eds) Perilous progress: technology as hazard. Westview, Boulder, Colorado, pp 91–123
7. Slovic P (1987) Perception of risk. Science, 236: 280–285
8. Szalay LB, Deese J (1978) Subjective meaning and culture: an assessment through word association. Erlbaum, Hillsdale, New Jersey
9. von Wartburg WP (1984) Drugs and the perception of risks. Swiss Pharma, 6 (No. 11a): 21–23

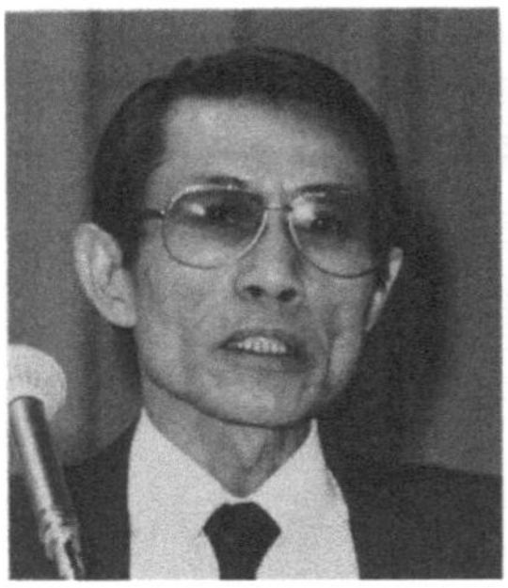

12. Risk Perception of Prescription Drugs: Report on Surveys in Japan

S. Fujino

Two surveys in 1987 and 1988 in Japan focused on the response by the general public and by physicians to many of the same questions concerning drugs and adverse drug reactions. In the public survey, a total of 1037 men and women aged between 20 and 69 filled out questionnaires in Tokyo and Osaka. A total of 1500 physicians in Japan took part in the other survey.

A major question in these surveys was whether doctors explained the effects of the drugs which they prescribed to patients. To this question, 38% of the general public answered "yes", compared to 31% who said "no", and 30% who replied "yes, if asked". Nearly 70% of the general public responded that physicians explained about the effects of drugs in some way. However, only 18% of the public said that their physicians explained about possible *adverse* drug reactions (ADRs), and 26% said, "yes, if asked". More than half (55%) reported that they received no explanation of ADRs from their physicians.

Physicians' responses to the same questions show a different perception. When asked whether they explained to patients about the drugs, 55% replied that they explained "to almost all patients", and 42% said that they explained about drugs "in some ways". In other words, physicians believed that they gave the required information about drugs to patients while the general public thought they did not receive enough information.

The content of explanations given by physicians was also examined in the surveys. Of the physicians, 83% said that their explanations centered on the efficacy of the drugs, 72% cited dosage and administration, and 68% primarily described possible ADRs. However, only 68% of the general public replied that they received an explanation on efficacy – a 15% difference from the physicians' responses. The perception gap is even greater with respect to ADRs: 44% of the general public said that they received an explanation – a 24% difference from the case with physicians.

The survey also asked whether patients complied with medication time, dose and frequency as recommended by their physician. Among the public, 35% replied that they "perfectly" complied with medication time, and 60% said "nearly perfectly". In addition, 43% said that they complied "perfectly" with their doctor's dose and frequency recommendations; 50% said "nearly perfectly". In response to the question of whether they took all the medication prescribed by physicians, only 21% replied affirmatively while 77% said that they stopped taking the medicine when they got better, "regardless of the remaining amount". It should be noted that over 40% of

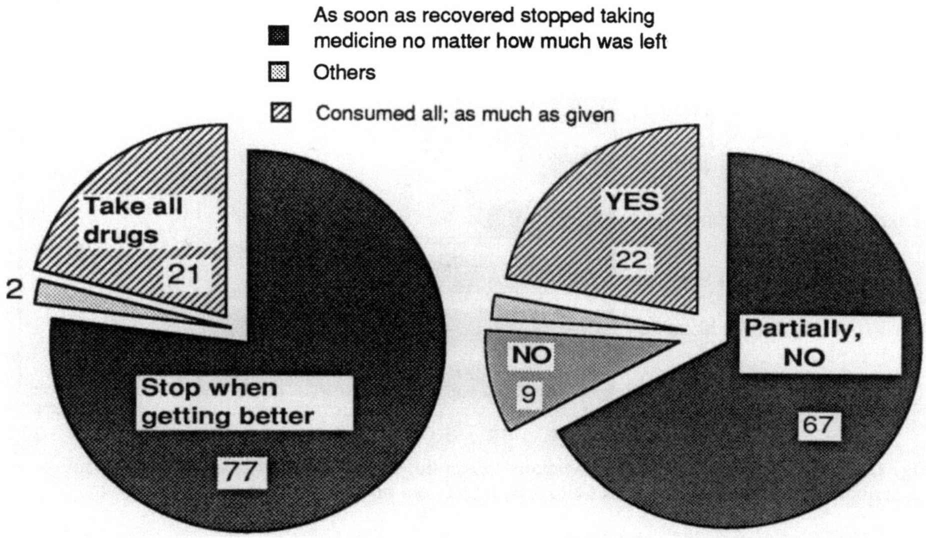

Fig. 12.1. Medication compliance: the public's reported response to directions for the intake of prescribed drugs. Figures represent percentages (n = 1037)

Fig. 12.2. Medication compliance: physicians' perceptions of patients' behavior towards the intake of prescribed drugs. Figures represent percentages in response to the question: "Do the patients follow doctors' directions?" (n = 1509)

the general public replied that they leave more than half of the prescribed medicine unused (Fig. 12.1). Among the physicians, 22% replied that most patients take medicine in compliance with directions, while 67% replied "partially not". Nine per cent of the physicians said that there was no compliance at all (Fig. 12.2). Thus, physicians recognized that the patients take medicine *more or less* in compliance with directions.

Both physicians and the general public were asked to describe patient behavior which resulted in the non-compliance (Fig. 12.3). Of the physicians, 72% said that they thought patients take medicine "capriciously", and 68% cited "erratic" behavior such as non-compliance in taking the correct daily dose, etc.; 59% of physicians said that patients suffered from incomplete medication because they stopped the intake of medicine during the treatment period. (This can be compared with the 77% of the general public who replied that they stopped taking medicine when they got better regardless of how much medicine remained.) The large percentage of patients who stopped taking medicine on their own judgement is one reason that physicians are often apprehensive about the risk of relapse or recurrence of symptoms.

Another part of the surveys covered prescription drug information. In Japan, only the directions for dosage and application are usually written on the package of prescribed medicine. The public and physicians were asked how they felt about this point. Whereas 75% of the general public said that they felt drug ingredients should

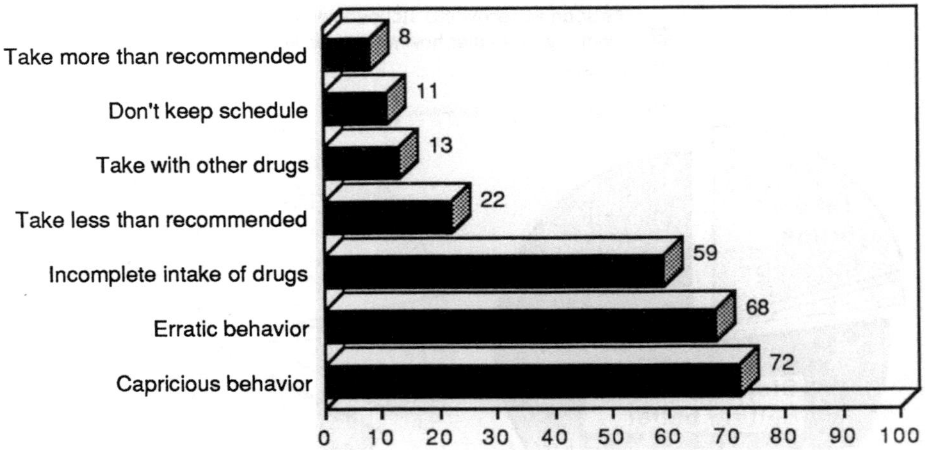

Fig. 12.3. Medication compliance: physicians' perceptions of patients' behavior towards the intake of prescribed drugs. Multiple responses allowed; figures are percentages

be included on the medicine package, only 20% of the physicians thought this to be needed (Fig. 12.4). And compared to the 83% of the general public who wanted drug information on efficacy, only 37% of physicians felt this necessary.

However, the two sets of responses resembled one another more closely with regard to the necessity of ADR information. The general public almost unanimously responded that ADR information was needed, indeed had priority over other information. A majority of the physicians, 62%, also felt ADR information should be included with prescription medicine.

In response to the question of how much ADR information physicians should give patients, physicians said that they should be careful in giving information unless very serious ADRs were anticipated. The reasons cited stressed that it is better not to make

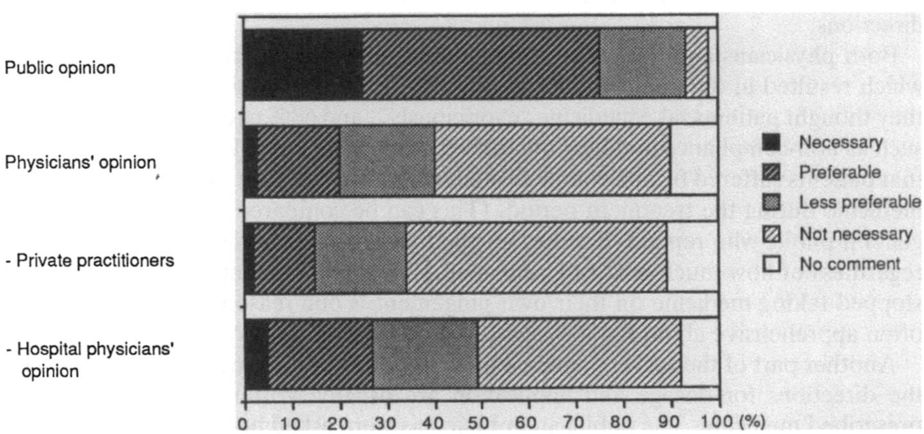

Fig. 12.4. Necessity for information on ingredients in drugs: perceptions of public and of physicians

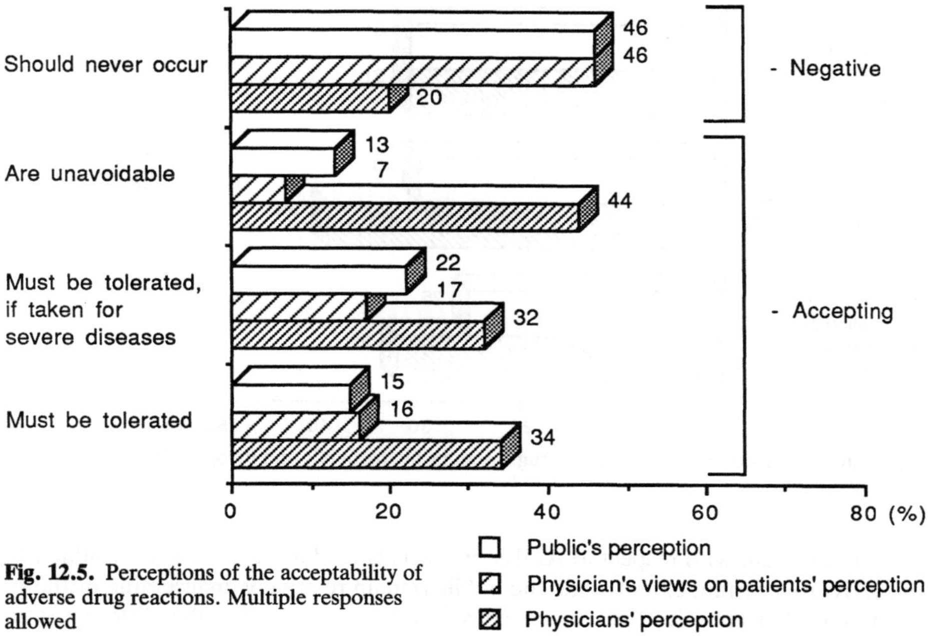

Fig. 12.5. Perceptions of the acceptability of adverse drug reactions. Multiple responses allowed

patients needlessly anxious about medicine, and that "it is not preferable to give shallow knowledge to patients". Those who answered this question concerning ADRs were allowed to give multiple answers (Fig. 12.5). Nearly half (46%) of the general public said, first of all, that ADRs "should never occur", and 20% of the physicians agreed with them. However, 44% of the physicians said that medicines do not always work selectively on the site of the disease, and that ADRs are in some ways unavoidable. Only 13% of the general public agreed with this. This indicates a large perception gap. A majority of both the physicians (77%) and the general public (54%) agreed that "ADRs may occur according to the patients' disease conditions".

The two groups were also asked about the perceived causes of ADRs (Fig. 12.6). Here, 39% of the general public and 30% of the physicians pointed to "incomplete systems for governmental approval and licensing". Identical percentages in the two groups – 31% – cited defects in the research and development system of the pharmaceutical industry. However, 32% of the general public replied that the cause of ADRs is inadequate drug information provided by physicians to the patients and/or improper dispensing. This compares with 25% of physicians who replied this way.

The survey included questions on preferences for Chinese herbal medicine as against chemically derived "Western" medicine. When asked which they would prefer to take, 32% of the general public favored Chinese herbal medicine, and 26% favored Western medicines; 32% responded "no interest", and 9% of the responders did not know. The overwhelmingly prevalent reason (90%) of responses cited for the choice of Chinese herbal medicine was that it has a lower incidence of ADRs.

In conclusion, the results of these surveys show perception gaps between what physicians and the general public in Japan believe about drugs and ADRs. This is

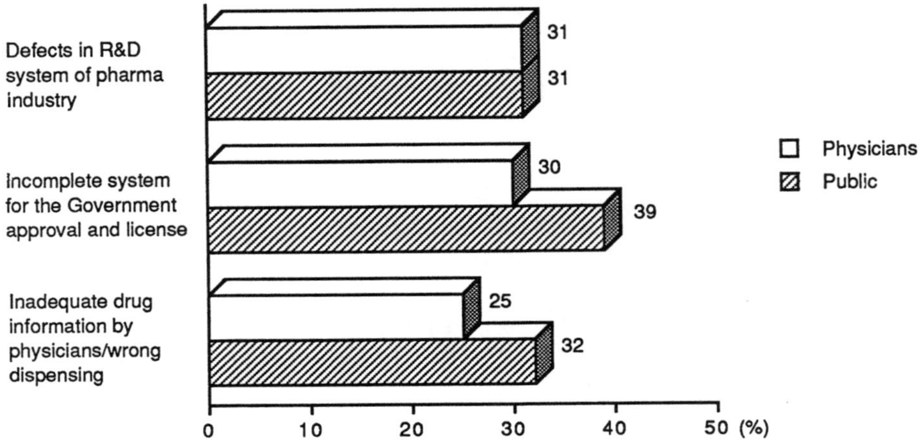

Fig. 12.6. Perceived causes of adverse drug reactions by the public and by physicians

particularly clear with respect to ADRs. Physicians tend to accept the unavoidability of ADRs to a certain extent while the public remain relatively unaccepting of them. Several background factors can be considered as reasons for the differences in perception. First, many social problems in Japan have been caused by drugs, such as thalidomide and those causing SMON. There have been many cases of evidently drug-induced suffering. Also, most ADR information concerned with drugs in Japan is related to risk, and almost nothing is written in the mass media about drug benefits.

It is very important to keep the general public adequately informed of the sincere efforts being made by industry, regulatory authorities and academic experts to improve drug safety.

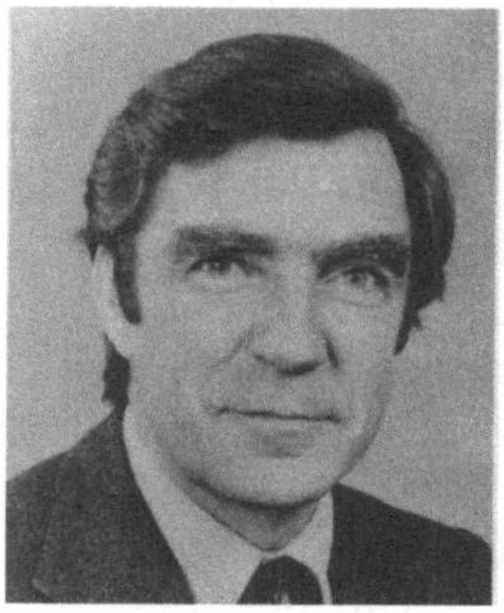

13. Scientific and Political Components of Regulatory Decision Making: General Considerations

G. Fülgraff

This paper does not focus on medicines but rather on certain factors in regulatory decision making regarding technologies and chemicals in general. It does not deal in particular with the often differing perceptions and judgments of issues by manufacturers and regulatory authorities or by industry scientists, managers, and the general public. Such questions are often addressed, issues are discussed, concerns expressed, interests demonstrated, and attempts made to understand the guiding rationale of the "other side" – with more or less success. Other speakers in this conference are better experienced to discuss these problems. Such discussion should be conducted without complaining, for example, about the irrational attitude or behavior of those who demand every possible effort be made to avoid incidents and diminish health risks at the work place in order to be in form to go skiing or hanggliding on the weekends. This brief presentation focuses rather on the relationship and some of the misunderstandings between the scientific and the nonscientific worlds concerning regulatory decisions.

Regulatory decisions on technologies and chemicals are based on estimates of risks (and benefits). Without going into detail, we can say that these estimates are derived from probabilistic, empirical, or experimental data. These estimates are more difficult to make

- the more complex a system is,
- the more interrelated the components of a system are;
- the less can be learned from previous accidents,
- and the farther away the experimental situation is from the "real world" or from the actual application.

This analysis and assessment – as opposed to evaluation – of risks and benefits is a process in which the scientific dimension dominates, and the work is carried out by expert scientists. It must be kept in mind, however, that even the assessment of risks is not a purely objective process which necessarily yields identical results when executed independently by two or more experts. Scientists and experts live, as do others, in their respective social environments, and they are exposed to the interests inherent in these. It is natural, human, and unavoidable that the institutional framework of a scientist's working conditions influences his reasoning and modifies his specific perspective. In view of this, in fact, it is amazing the degree to which analyses and estimates are consistent across groups of scientists.

The data on risks and benefits must be *evaluated* prior to regulatory action. It is evident that these evaluations of scientific data go beyond scientific grounds. Social value judgments are involved. Whenever the questions asked include those such as "How do we want to live?" they are political ones. And questions of this type are involved when data of risk/benefit analyses are evaluated with a view to possible alternative regulatory reactions. Thus, the evaluation of risks versus benefits is a process in which the social and political dimension prevails. Scientific advice, however, is needed in the evaluation.

The two processes, analysis and evaluation, cannot be completely separated. Scientists involved in these processes in preparation for regulatory decisions must nevertheless recognize that their professional prerogative ends with the stage of analysis, and they should accept that they are no longer at an advantage due to their expertise and scientific rationality when it comes to making value judgments. Instead, these judgments should be based upon the broadest possible consensus in a society regarding the acceptance of specific risks.

The relative role of scientific versus political competence may differ according to the subject under consideration, its importance, and its generality. In the case of pharmaceuticals, the scientific component predominates whereas in the case of nuclear energy, for example, the political component must be of greater importance. In neither case, however, can either component be neglected. It is therefore difficult to understand why "lay" representatives should be excluded from committees charged with the analysis and evaluation of medicines. It can, in fact, be very helpful for regulators to listen to scientific experts explaining the key criteria of their reasoning to the lay public.

For many scientists rationality means following their own criteria and value scales. Persons with conflicting judgments are then considered to be reacting, by definition, in an irrational or emotional way. This is a very dangerous attitude because it sets scientific expertise apart from the social consensus of society. A nonemotional discussion of risks fails to recognize that society has difficulty coping with man-made risks. The question thus arises, whether in the long term, human thinking and feeling must adjust itself to new risks (which is usually called a rational attitude and behavior), or whether society should cease producing risks with which its members cannot cope. Philosophers nowadays work on theories of different types of rationality. Thus, one can criticize specifically scientific-technical rationality without renouncing rationality per se. Exhaustive information on the complexities in many fields of modern science and technology overburden the individual, and when a purely rational handling of and coping with all problems necessarily fails, the result may be an escape into emotional reactions. No one can be blamed for this. Perception and acceptance of risks are not scientific reactions and do not follow natural laws but are determined rather by social and cultural factors.

Finally, it must be acknowledged that a general view of risks does not in itself produce individual acceptance of risks. It is often irrelevant to the individual's acceptance of a risk whether scientists' estimates are of an order of magnitude greater or smaller. For such acceptance, other criteria are of greater importance – such as personal experience, voluntary exposure, or immediate benefit. Studies indicate, on the other hand, that for experts the low incidence of a specific risk is a high-ranking criterion, whereas for the lay public the potential danger counts more.

The preparing of regulatory decisions must consider cultural and social determinants of the perception of risks. Hence, the evaluation of scientific data on risks and benefits can yield different results and lead to different regulatory measures in different societies and even in the same society at different times. I know that many of my colleagues still reject these postulates, but I believe these to be rear-guard conflicts – if you will excuse this use of military language.

The experts involved in analysis and evaluation of risks are usually researchers. This signifies not only competence and knowledge but also involvement, diminished distance, and reduced ability to critique. How, for example, could the begetter of a product or technique ever be expected to condemn his "child"? And products and technologies usually have many such "fathers". The lay public has a good appreciation of these difficulties in its acceptance of the knowledge, but not the value judgments, of expert scientists.

In a way, expert scientists must be regarded as constituting an interest group. The products or techniques which they or their colleagues have been working on, they wish to see realized, sold, and used. This is the final objective of their work. Hence, it is not surprising that scientists are usually more affirmative than the general public in judging the acceptability of a given risk.

Another source of misunderstanding between experts and others is the way in which experts talk about and handle the different components of risks. They do not always discriminate in a sufficiently clear and outspoken manner between determinable and nondeterminable risks.

In the case of chemicals, for example, the determinable risk can be estimated using all available sources of knowledge from animal experiments as well as from human exposure including the relation of concentration or dose level and observed effects, the profile of the effects, the dose- or concentration-effect relation, the dose- or concentration-frequency relation, the fate of the substance of exposed persons, etc. There remains, nevertheless, a nondeterminable risk comprising all those components which cannot be quantified or even exactly described, but which are part of the overall risk. The determinable risk must be distinguished from the nondeterminable risk because the two are essentially different and must be judged differently, even though it is possible that aspects of the nondeterminable risk in future may be attributed to the determinable risk. Elimination of the nondeterminable risk is by definition not possible. It can be reduced by significant safety factors, but it cannot be eliminated.

I believe that scientists and experts will gain trust among the public for their capability to assess risks, the more they express themselves clearly on the necessary limitations of their knowledge. By its nature, nondeterminable risk is open to very subjective interpretations and judgments by experts as well as by the public. The expectation of experts that this risk is rather low is based on the experience that grave mistakes have been rare. But this expectation has no predictive value and is therefore not very convincing to the public. The acceptance of risks to which people are involuntarily exposed depends largely on an honest and open discussion on these risks, their nature, and the main factors which contribute to them; in these discussions the public's uneasiness should not be regarded as an emotional reaction which therefore does not need to be seriously considered.

Among the many factors which can contribute to the nondeterminable risk of chemicals (including pharmaceuticals) and which are of varying importance are the following:
- The nonoccurrence of effects in biological systems cannot, strictly speaking, be proven.
- Only the effects which are looked for can be discovered; others may be disregarded.
- The ability to observe effects is a function of the sensitivity of the available systems of observation and investigation.
- Effects due to chemicals, be they environmental chemicals, chemicals in the workplace, or medicines, can be detected neither from animal experiments nor from epidemiological studies with a sufficient degree of probabilitiy when the same or similar effects can also be provoked by other causes or may even occur "spontaneously".
- One must bear in mind, even if it appears banal, that statistical analyses allow only statements of probability, not proof, of causal correlations.
- Rare effects are likely to be overlooked; even if recorded, they cannot be quantified. The failure of the "mega-mouse experiment" demonstrated the technical and structural limitations of very large animal experiments.
- The extrapolation from animal experiments to humans has its pitfalls; safety factors are applied mainly to reduce this uncertainty.
- Humans are exposed to many different substances, which makes it impossible to consider or to make reasonable assumptions about all possible interactions.
- For many important reactions no experimental models are available which could allow an ex ante assessment – a typical example is allergy.
- The methodology to validate subjective factors and impairments is insufficiently developed.
- It is not possible to detect systematically and in a general way persons or groups of persons for whom exposure constitutes a higher risk.

This short enumeration of factors included in the nondeterminable risk is not intended to be complete but rather illustrative.

To conclude, it is probably useful to look at the behavior of scientists in two different situations: when they make risk/benefit judgments for themselves, and when they are talking about scientific and technological developments in fields which are not their own. For the former, it would be very interesting, for example, to have data on the prescribing habits of medical doctors when treating their relatives or themselves as compared to that in the treatment of their patients. Regarding the latter situation, one could consider the case of nuclear power plant managers who are worried about developments in modern synthetic biology or that of genetic engineers who are uneasy about the safety of nuclear energy; both groups may complain about modern medicine and about adverse reactions to pharmaceuticals.

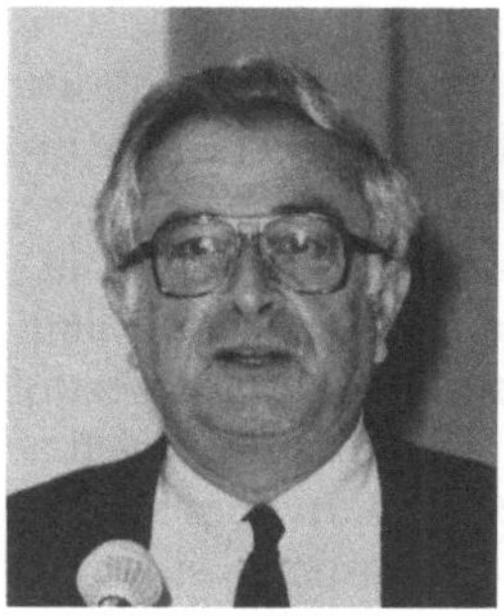

14. Scientific and Political Components of Regulatory Decision Making: The United States Experience

L. Lasagna

Regulatory decisions are affected by both scientific and political considerations. While these components are not necessarily independent of each other, it is nevertheless useful to consider them separately.

Scientific Components

The most important scientifically based regulatory decisions about medicines have, of course, to do with the safety and efficacy of marketed drugs. For a new chemical entity to achieve approval for marketing requires the accumulation of substantial evidence, from animal and human studies, that the chemical (or biological product) can provide potential health benefits of sufficient magnitude that the potential adverse effects (both qualitatively and quantitatively) pose an acceptable risk.

Put as a generality, this principle seems simplicity itself. But, as this audience knows all too well, the process of reaching a judgment on this point depends not only on the nature and volume of the data submitted to the regulatory agency, but on the inevitable subjective weighing, by fallible human beings, of the quality and quantity of the evidence and the projection from that evidence, gathered in situations quite unlike ordinary medical practice, to the universe of patients who will be treated by the prescribing physicians, and an educated guess to the effect that, if the drug is used as directed, it will do much more good than harm. Considering the fact that the preregistration analysis is one of *groups* of patients, and that postregistration usage focuses on *individuals*, it is in a sense surprising that projections are as good as they are.

History reminds us that regulatory demands for the data base on which approval rests have varied enormously over the years. In the United States, for example, proof of efficacy was not required by statute until 1962, although there had previously been de facto examination of the evidence of efficacy to allow toxicity data to be sensibly evaluated. The Supreme Court had, actually, in 1911 decided that efficacy was, in fact, only a matter of opinion and therefore did not deserve legal recognition.

These changing regulatory requirements are related to both the state of the art and the reigning regulatory dogma. Today the regulatory agencies in most countries rely heavily on modern randomized controlled clinical trials and certain principles of experimental design and statistical analysis that were borrowed (at least in part) from agricultural research. The almost invariable need, in the United States, for *replicate* trials is related in part to the principle that repetition of research findings is a traditional basis for acceptance by the scientific community, but this is based primarily on regulatory rules rather than on explicit demands by the scientific establishment or by the governing statute or the legislative history of the 1962 Amendments.

The preoccupation with controlled trials is at times quite inappropriate. There is, for instance, no clear scientific justification for double-blind randomized controlled clinical trials if one wants to determine whether a chemical has useful antineoplastic activity, as opposed to making *comparative* statements about the efficiacy of such a chemical. There is also considerable controversy as to whether modern approval of anticancer drugs should be contingent on the achievement only of shrinkage in tumor mass or on complete clinical remissions, or should require evidence of prolongation of life and improved quality of life, end points vastly more difficult to quantify [1].

While it would be difficult to conceive of a more fundamental scientific canon of pharmacology than the dose-response curve, adequate exploration of dose-response is often lacking in preregistration studies. The result has been, at times, the marketing of drugs at recommended doses either higher or lower than optimal. Hydrochlorothiazide and captopril are two examples of drugs originally introduced at doses that in retrospect were grossly too high (eightfold!). Failures of estimation of this sort can, of course, both needlessly stigmatize a medicine and increase its cost to consumers.

Even when national statutes specifically bar the withholding of registration on the basis of relative efficacy, in fact a chemical may fail to achieve registration if the judgment (not an easy one) made by regulators is that it is not uniquely useful and significantly less safe than older drugs.

In assessing safety, the specific animal species studied, the numbers of experimental animals, the dose levels employed, the variables measured, and the duration of the experiments are quite arbitrary matters. Walker, for example, has amassed data from industrial laboratories that suggest strongly that we carry out more animal toxicity tests for longer periods of times than we need to. The result is unnecessary waste of time and resources, with little scientific benefit [2].

There is also considerable evidence [3] that teratogenicity studies abound in false positives and false negatives. Carcinogenicity tests in animals are performed routinely despite the fact that their relevance to humans has never been fully evaluated, and that they add hundreds of thousands of dollars and 3 years of testing to a drug's developmental history. (Do we really need carcinogenicity tests on anticancer drugs?)

The subjective nature of the decision-making process has been beautifully illustrated by Leighton [4]. His company submitted the same new drug application to seven different regulatory agencies. "Deficiencies" varied from agency to agency, indicating that a "deficiency" resides as much with the agency as with the application, and that accelerating reviews of applications is not simply a matter of eliminating obvious deficiencies.

The history of bioequivalence standards testifies eloquently to the need to change requirements as evidence accumulates that older standards are inadequate. At first, in the United States, a manufacturer had only to make dosage forms that contained the proper chemical in proper amount. Later, disintegration-time assays were added, then in vitro dissolution rates, and finally actual absorption, distribution, and elimination studies in healthy volunteers. Now there is evidence that results in healthy individuals may not always predict what will happen in the sick, so that we can anticipate still further changes in the standard techniques.

The advent of biotechnology products will probably force the adoption of new standards in quality control, as one worries about loss in potency due to alterations in the dimensional conformation of proteins much larger and more complex than conventional drug molecules, and about new problems (e. g., of immunogenicity) from cell culture impurities.

Statistical analysis has become a way of life in drug regulation, although it is not clear that we are always wisely applying statistical principles. For 20 years statistical journals have pointed out the limits of formal hypothesis testing in the analysis of experimental data, but regulators (and editors!) continue to worship at this statistical shrine [5]. Alpha-levels, arbitrarily set, have become like religious dogma. "Intent-to-treat" analyses are considered by the United States Food and Drug Administration (FDA) as the "least biased" type of analysis, despite the fact that such analyses may count patients who have never received the drug (or have even received *another* drug!).

There is a belief among many regulatory statisticians that analyses of data that were not planned at the start of the experiment serve at best for "hypothesis generating". Of interest are the strong opinions against this principle voiced by some NIH statistical giants as far back as 1965 [6]. Let me quote one:

"Of course a re-examination in the light of results of the assumptions on which the pre-observational partition of the sample space was based would be regarded in some circles as bad statistics. It would, however, be widely regarded as good science. I do not believe that anything that is good science can be bad statistics, and ... (I) hope that there are no statisticians so inflexible as to decline to analyze an honest body of scientific data simply because it fails to conform to some favored theoretical scheme. If there are such, however, clinical trials, in my opinion, are not for them."

The above quotation of Jerome Cornfield is one that I favor, because I believe that we need to do *more* subset analyses of data, not fewer. We should always try to determine whether our experimental results suggest patient factors that predispose either to benefit or to harm. One obvious variable of importance always deserving of separate analysis is compliance. Failure to take medicine can, to be sure, either cause a drug to fail or reflect failure, i. e., result from the patient's or physician's perception (perhaps correct) that the drug is either ineffective or toxic. But consider the correlation, presented in Table 14.1, between amount of drug ingested in a cholestyramine trial and the effect on serum cholesterol and risk of coronary heart diesease [10]. These are, I submit, impressive data far superior to "average" performance in communicating to physicians and patients the potential benefit of compliance. (The figures are, by the way, contained in the United States package insert, agreed to both by the manufacturer and the FDA.)

Table 14.1. Cholestyramine, serum cholesterol, and coronary heart disease

Packets taken daily	Serum cholesterol lowering	Decrease in CHD risk
0–2	4.4%	10.9%
2–5	11.5%	26.1%
5–6	19.0%	39.3%

Science also tells us that knowledge about a drug is never complete, and that new information about benefit or harm may accrue years after a drug's original approval. There is no way to acquire all this information prior to marketing, so that we clearly need to keep improving our postregistration efforts to detect new findings at the earliest possible opportunity.

We also know that good drugs may be poorly used and may thus be unfairly blamed for faults that lie with prescribers or patients. Detection or prevention of such malprescribing cannot be done by central fiat or monitoring; it requires local action, such as might be invoked by a clinical pharmacologist or clinical pharmacist monitoring the quality of drug usage in a hospital. I have proposed that such monitoring be a prerequisite to accreditation of hospitals. Scientific requirements also apply to attempts to insure "good manufacturing practice" or "good laboratory practice," although once again there are inevitably value judgments made by regulators in their demands.

If human judgments are inevitably involved in regulation, how can we improve the quality of these judgments? One way is to train adequately those who review data submitted to regulatory agencies. There is little in the training of most health professionals that prepares them to assess such data, and therefore they need to be trained in such matters as protocol design, statistics, epidemiology, the realities of clinical trials, etc. The same applies to statisticians, who need to be trained to interact with biologists and health professionals.

Even so, however, we must anticipate that consensus will often be difficult to achieve, even among people of experience and good will. It is depressing but not surprising that the EEC has been so unsuccessful in harmonizing drug regulatory *decisions*, in contrast with the at least partial harmonization of general *documentation procedures*.

Political Components

Politicians not infrequently have an impact on drug regulation, for a variety of reasons. To begin with, health news is of great interest to the public. Elected officials want their constituent voters to feel that they worry about both the health of the public's bodies and minds and the health of their pocketbooks. Unexpected toxicity and the withdrawal of a drug from the market for this reason may therefore cause heads to roll in regulatory agencies or in ministries of health. This phenomenon can engender a paralytic regulatory "fear of error." Thalidomide offers a prime example of the importance of the phenomenon, but there have been more recent examples.

Political pressure can also arise from public health needs. The AIDS epidemic is a dramatic instance. This modern plague has created understandable anxiety, a less defensible hysteria, and a demand for prompt solutions. But the challenges are formidable. Consider the problems in coming up with an AIDS vaccine:

1. We are dealing with a human retrovirus, not an ordinary microbe.
2. The disease is characterized by immunoparalysis, so that the presence of antibodies does not necessarily indicate protection.
3. There is no adequate animal model, and the selection of vaccine candidates is chancy at best.

4. The possibility for harm (social or biologic) to vaccination trial volunteers is very real.

Pressures also come from such quarters as patient advocacy groups, disease-oriented foundations, consumer advocates, and scientific bureaucrats (in government or academe) who are competing for shrinking resources or who are evangelists for certain therapeutic or research programs.

The public communications media can be either helpful or mischievous. Their main motivation often seems to be popularity with their readers or viewers, which is often not consonant with a balanced presentation of facts and problems. Many a scientist and regulator has had occasion to rue the decision to appear on a sensationalist television program and to suffer from lurid coverage and unscrupulous editing and splicing of camera footage.

The mounting pressures to contain the cost of health care are leading to constraints on drug prices and hence on new drug research. Third World advocates often seem to be antiprofit and antipatents in their attitudes, despite the fact that most of our pharmacopeia is the result of capitalistically driven research. In this regard, it is of interest that a recent study by our center at Tufts found that about 50% of the medicines in the latest World Health Organization (WHO) Essential Drug List were "me-too" drugs, i.e., not the first drug in a given therapeutic class. About 20% of the WHO drugs have "follow-on" indications listed, i.e., not the indication originally approved at the time of marketing. Hence if industry had not pursued molecular modification and had not pursued post-approval research for new indications, the WHO list would be much shorter and poorer. While drug needs are not the same in developing and developed countries, untreatable diseases are a problem for all. AIDS patients are dying as pitifully in Africa and in Central and South America as in Amsterdam, London, San Francisco, and New York.

Animal rights advocates are forcing scientists to reevaluate whether animal testing is being performed improperly or unnecessarily. An honest analysis of such testing and the elimination of needless research would be a boon; the hazard is that such activists may convince politicians to ban *all* animal research as cruel and immoral.

"Bioethicists" continue to ask searching questions about the conduct of human research. Changes in research procedures and informed consent requirements have certainly slowed down (and occasionally prevented) certain kinds of research. The ethical benefits of such scrutiny have been substantial, but there are also losses from the hampering of research.

The legal profession, especially in the United States, is shaping the kinds of information provided to physicians and patients and affecting both medical practice and industrial budgets by the threat of litigation for damages, either real or putative. We have recently reviewed the "Bendectin saga" and concluded that there will never be another drug marketed in the United States for treating the nausea and vomiting of pregnancy – a direct consequence of the many law suits against the manufacturer of Bendectin [7].

Finally, there are cultural pressures that affect drug regulation. Countries with continuing interest among the public and certain health professionals in "traditional" or "homeopathic" or "anthroposophic" remedies may find it difficult to apply the same regulatory criteria to these unorthodox remedies as they apply to conventional medicines.

A variant of this theme was discussed in our paper on Depo-Provera, an injectable contraceptive that received completely opposite recommendations from expert committees in the United Kingdom and the United States, explained, we believe, by the different regulatory philosophies of the two countries [8].

Conclusion

The lessons that we can draw are the following:

1. Whether dealing with scientific or political components of drug regulation, risk-benefit considerations are often involved in the decision.
2. One searches in vain for any formal calculus used to make risk-benefit decisions in the area of drug regulation, and regulators will usually decide that a medicine is "safe enough" or "not safe enough" in a fashion that seems unrelated to any explicit risk-benefit formula.
3. Determinants of regulatory decisions vary in type and importance from country to country and from time to time.
4. Regulatory agencies tend to have, as their charge or remit, the protection or safeguarding of public health, not its *promotion*. (In the United States, there is a striking difference between the charge to the FDA and that to the Federal Aviation Agency.)
5. The public rarely has information about the costs, risks, and benefits of technologies presented in such a way as to "illuminate the available choices" and "permit individuals to reach informed judgments" [9]. In this regard, government, industry, the health professions, and the public media share the guilt.
6. Public perceptions of risk often seem unrelated to the actual magnitude of risk. A nuclear disaster in Chernobyl overshadows the risk of the mining and burning of coal or other fossil fuels (or, in the United States, even the risk of handguns!). One terrorist attack in an airport may temporarily cause millions of tourists to ruin their travel plans. With regard to drugs, the public seems more concerned about the risks from drugs than about the harm from not taking indicated drugs or the harm that ensues if we do not successfully devise needed new medicines. If programs such as RAD-AR can redress this imbalance, we shall all be better off.

References

1. Wittes RE (1987) Antineoplastic agents and FDA regulations: square pegs for round holes? Cancer Treat Rep 71: 795–806
2. Walker SR (1986) A retrospective analysis of chronic toxicity case studies on pharmaceutical compounds. In: Walker SR, Dayan AD (eds) Long-term animal studies: their predictive value for man. MTP, Lancaster, pp 53–62
3. Lasagna L (1987) Predicting human drug safety from animal studies: current issues. J Toxicol Sci 12: 439–450
4. Lasagna L, Bearn AG (eds) (1987) Innovation and acceleration in clinical drug development, MEDAC, Medical Advisory Coucil, June 9–10, 1986, Raven, New York
5. Lasagna L (1987) On assuring pharmacotherapeutic progress in the 21st century. Br J Clin Pharmacol 23: 659–665

6. Cutler SJ, Greenhouse SW, Cornfield J, et al. (1966) The role of hypothesis testing in clinical trials. National Institutes of Health Biometrics Seminar, Maryland, June, 1965. J Chronic Dis 19: 857–882
7. Barash CI, Lasagna L (1987) The Bendectin saga: "voluntary" discontinuation. J Clin Res Drug Dev 1: 277–292
8. Richard BW, Lasagna L (1987) Drug regulation in the United States and the United Kingdom: the Depo-Provera story. Ann Intern Med 106: 886–891
9. Winsten JA (1985) Science and the media: the boundaries of truth. Health Aff (Millwood) 4(1): 5–23
10. Physicians' Desk Reference (1987) Medical Economics Co., Oradell, New York

15. Summary of Part II: Presentations and Discussions

Speakers at the beginning of the session underscored the theme that risk analysis alone is insufficient, that there must be appreciation of both perception and communication of risk. They then discussed the limitations of available data on the safety of prescription drugs: limits both of studies to evaluate efficacy and of the reporting of voluntary postmarketing adverse drug reactions. Attention focused on computer-based medical record linkage systems which could provide rapid access to the information needed to answer safety questions about new drugs. Currently, several medical data bases exist, but their cumulative size is too small to provide answers to critical drug risk questions. (Systems including about ten million people are required for safety studies of newly marketed drugs.) Other problems of current medical data systems are confidentiality, cost, technical organization, and immediate access to records.

The scenario of a theoretical drug problem was examined: a drug which, after four randomized controlled trials, has been successfully on the market for 10 years comes

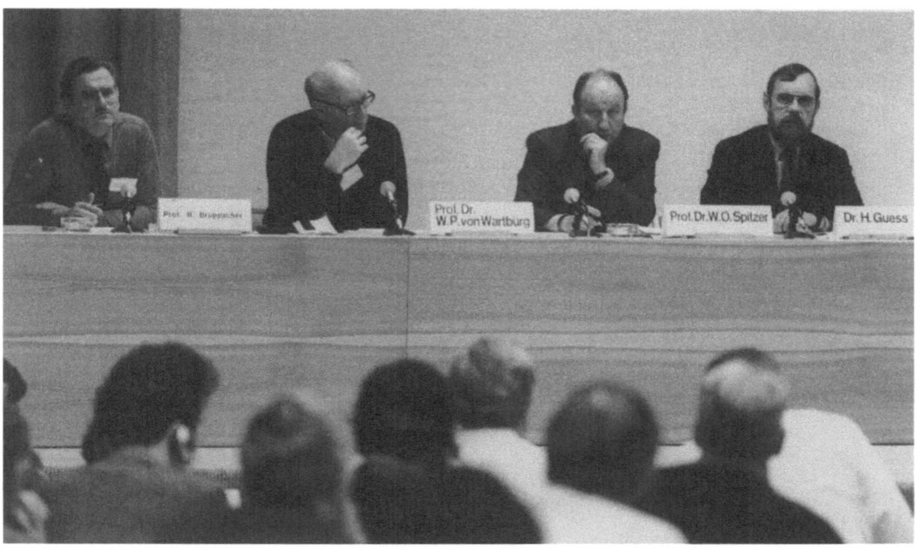

under fire after a substantial number of adverse reports and for causing a new syndrome. The audience was asked to look at possible studies and at methodology which have been used in evaluating the drug.

Varying strategies (including cohort studies and case-control studies) were reviewed as well as the types of biases which may affect the data. Reactions to an apparent cluster of significant clinical events – especially adverse reactions – were discussed, and the distinctions between association and causation were made. Guidelines for scientific admissability of evidence, including biostatistical considerations, were also examined. It was pointed out that a critical situation develops when there is a conflict within a pharmaceutical company between marketing and safety.

In the second part of the program on benefit/risk analysis and appraisal, a representative of an American pharmaceutical firm reviewed how it had successfully confronted charges by a consumer group that one of its drugs was unsafe. The consumer group had filed an imminent hazard petition with the Food and Drug Administration in February 1986, and in July of that year, after hearings had been held, the petition was denied and the drug cleared. The presentation examined the critical roles of formal epidemiological studies and the availability of pharmacoepidemiological resources in demonstrating that the petition was without merit. The use of medical data bases – by both the firm and the FDA – was critical to quickly providing the needed data on the drug and adverse drug reaction reports. The impact of the public controversy over the drug was also carefully examined in the presentation.

Scientific and political components of regulatory decision making were explained separately and examined to show how they are interrelated. Scientific components include evaluation of human data relevant to the safety and efficacy of medicines, "state-of-the-art" techniques used in the evaluations, dose-response relationships, bioequivalency standards, statistical practices, etc. Political factors include the value to elected officials of publicity about drug safety, efficacy, and cost; the media; desires of patient advocacy groups; economic pressures; ethical concerns and litigation. For most of these factors, risk-benefit calculations are either explicit or implicit, although a formal calculus is almost never involved.

In an effort to determine what can be learned from drug safety problems, an analysis was made of past and present drug safety issues. Patterns emerged which show types of behavior – especially by the pharmaceutical companies – which apparently increase the vulnerability of a particular drug and possibly also the likelihood that it may be withdrawn from the market. These include exaggerated claims, misleading or inconsistent product information, and failure to react properly or quickly when new adverse reactions are reported. A combination of these factors can be particularly devastating. The key actors who influence the final decision about a drug safety issue are the pharmaceutical manufacturers, university scientists, members of the medical profession, regulators, politicians, and the media. Interdisciplinary and cooperative efforts which recognize the public's interest in the area, and which allow for public participation can offer a realistic chance of improvement in communication and understanding.

During the course of the discussion, the question was raised as to the desirability, feasibility, and ethics of pharmaceutical companies cooperating financially to subsidize development of medical records systems, especially where common interests in drugs are concerned. It was agreed that it would be highly desirable for pharmaceutical companies financially to subsidize medical records systems, but the problem of how to do this remained unresolved.

It was generally acknowledged that most pharmaceutical companies support medical records linkage systems, and many contribute financially to them, but support by the industry needs to be far greater and better organized. Currently, the pharmaceutical industry's contributions to these data base systems are a fraction of what it costs to run them; the real costs are not borne by industry.

Attention was drawn by one participant to the particular hallmarks of pharmacoepidemiology – as compared to epidemiology in general. For some, he said, its distinguishing characteristic is the search for rare situations, a search which could only be quick and effective if large data bases were used. On the other hand, he added, although pharmacoepidemiology studies drug effects, this focus in itself may be too narrow. The problems lie in the understanding of diseases and patient populations and a whole spectrum of study conditions and limitations.

In contrast with clinical research, pharmacoepidemiology covers the causal links between an event, exposure factors, and drugs, as well as unexpected benefits such as improving quality of life. An important hallmark is its aid in improving the clinical decision with respect to individual patients. But pharmacoepidemiology is probably most critical in aiding the improvement of public health decisions where the entire community is at risk.

The statistical question remains, just how likely is it that a risk will be detected? Risk is usually very difficult to detect by controlled clinical trials. How many cases must there be before one has a better than fifty-fifty chance of predicting risk? Not all adverse drug reaction cases are observed, and pharmacoepidemiology has its limits, which are not only statistical but also due to intrinsic factors such as the properties of the drug and the way in which the drug is used by patients and doctors. Unless one takes into account all the probabilities and other factors, one is unlikely to predict the possibility of drug risk.

One speaker suggested that companies should make decisions based on what they consider to be the best business, moral, and ethical judgment and *then* consult lawyers to find out what the risks are of following these decisions. He observed that lawyers are generally risk aversive, and their advice would be for great caution – which may not necessarily be in best general interest of the company.

Questions that the public has regarding risk assessment by the pharmaceutical companies were discussed. It was pointed out that there are risks that are perceived by management at various times in a drug's life. The public wants to know, when management makes decisions about marketing these drugs, how is risk assessment involved in the decision? If a company markets a product, knowing there are risks involved, is it balancing known risks against sales decisions, etc.? The public also wants to know, when drug risk is considered, whether there is any idea of what is likely to happen to people taking the drug in question. It was suggested that an independent panel be set up with worldwide experts, and that this panel monitor new drugs and provide unbiased opinions.

Another person in the discussion strongly recommended that members of a committee on drug safety should be concerned simply with the welfare of consumers.

More than one speaker said that it is wrong to make decisions on the safety of drugs in secrecy, and that the public should not tolerate such a situation.

It was described as a paradox that, while a very carefully selected group of people are chosen for clinical trials, as soon as a drug is approved, it is given to persons who bear very little resemblance to those who used it in the trials. The circumstances in which a drug is used in reality are frequently dissimilar to those which existed in the trials.

In conclusion, it was pointed out that the pharmaceutical industry should not lose touch with the public, should not forget the obvious question that the public wants answered: "Is this drug doing undue harm: yes or no?" The pharmaceutical industry should give thought in advance of a problem to how to deal with questions quickly, sensibly, and without becoming defensive. Communication between industry and the public should not be couched in jargon and technical terms but in straightforward language which is easily understandable. Misunderstandings result only in higher anxiety levels.

Part III

Current Challenges

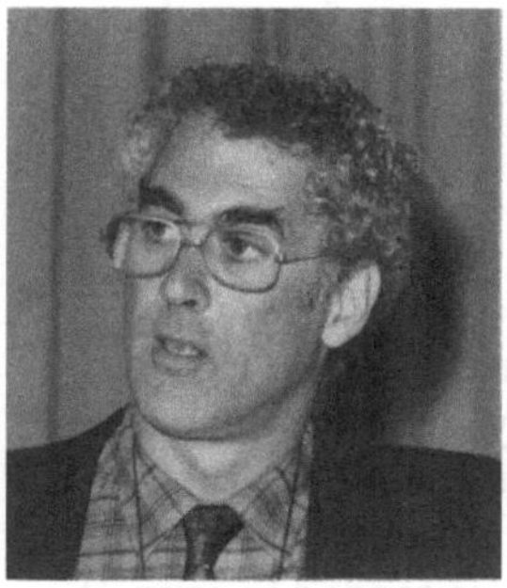

16. Professional Drug Information: A Consumer Perspective

C. MEDAWAR

Introduction

This paper takes up where an earlier discussion of "failings of the pharmaceutical industry" left off [1]. That earlier paper – which like this one was intended not so much to offer criticism as to explain how and why it arises – emphasised the following main points:

1. In spite of, and to some extent because of, the contributions the industry has made to world health, there are still substantial grounds for criticism of some of its activities.
2. The industry has tended to react over-defensively to such criticism which has at times "caused it to misjudge the opposition it faces and therefore to respond quite inappropriately to it". I suggested, for example, that the industry's response to criticism from the consumer movement has tended to strengthen the consumer movement, but to weaken the industry's cause.
3. The industry cannot effectively counter the criticism it gets by attending to its image rather than to matters of substance. One of several reasons for suggesting this is that image-building tends to have a self-intoxicating effect, causing people within the industry to overlook the need to attend to what is wrong.
4. If the industry does not clearly understand the difference between "right" and "wrong" – at least as this is perceived by consumer and other critics – it will always find it difficult to get it "right".

Each of these four propositions embodies the idea that this "power failure" originates from within the pharmaceutical industry and is mainly the result of industry action or inaction. It follows that the power failure can be expected to continue until the industry decides to do something about it. For a start, it has to be clearly recognised that the industry cannot control its own destiny.

The somewhat precarious nature of the business of making drugs – which involves relatively high-risk and very long-term investment and decision-making – makes it easy to understand why the industry should seek such a high degree of control over what it perceives as it own affairs. But the fact is that the industry's products and performance are also intimately to do with human destiny, which is something people want to control themselves. Thus, the more the industry tries to control its own destiny, the more distanced it may become from the true consumers of its products – and therefore the more likely it is to fail.

Nature and Control of power

A premise of this analysis is that the power which the pharmaceutical industry has – which in essence derives quite legitimately from its capacity to transform human health and less legitimately because of our dependence on this – has a destructive as well as a constructive side to it. On the one hand, the industry's power has allowed it to develop better medicines. On the other hand, this power has also tended to corrupt – for reasons which have less to do with the character of the industry than with the nature of power.

The dose-response relationship, between these two was articulated by Lord Acton in the memorable statement: "All power corrupts, but absolute power corrupts absolutely". This does not only apply to individuals. It probably applies even more to organisations, especially when the individual members of these organisations are strongly bound to corporate goals and/or relatively far-distanced from the end consumers of its services and products. Both apply of the pharmaceutical industry.

It is generally recognised that checks and balances are needed to ensure that power is used wisely and well. For example, in a system of democratic government, checks and balances are mainly provided by means of an institutionalised opposition: while the power of business organisations is subject to the discipline of the market place. However, the pharmaceutical industry is significantly different. Conventional systems of checks and balances do not operate, mainly because of the diminished and very dependent status of the consumers of its products. Consumers of medicines have traditionally been expected to be "compliant", to be grateful, but not too demanding, and never to be so silly as to assume that they are entitled to perfect safety. They have generally been told what to do and what is good for them by experts whose approach was "that only a few people knew certain facts and that the majority of the population knew little or held the wrong views" [2]. Patients (otherwise often referred to as "poor things") have been in almost no position to provide checks and balances over the pharmaceutical industry. That function has been left to government and to the medical profession instead.

However, I suggest that neither government nor the medical profession has been able to provide the discipline the industry needs, because both have to some extent been compromised by taking a share of the industry's wealth and power. Governments have been compromised, if not through the operation of informal systems of the kind documented by Braithwaite [3], then through their dependence on the industry's wealth, including its earnings of foreign exchange. In times of trouble, the industry has always been been ready to point out what government might lose if its wealth was withdrawn and shared elsewhere – but most governments probably need little reminding.

At the same time, the medical profession has been compromised both because of its dependence on the industry's products as a major source of its own power – also because of the industry's increasing sponsorship of science and through the operation of generous if not lavish reward systems [4].

In relation to professional drug information, the medical profession has two main things to answer for. One is that it has come to tolerate and also to contribute to unacceptably low standards of information about drugs and their effects. The other is that the profession has consistently and quite unreasonably denied that the provision of such information could possibly have encouraged it to depart from the high standards of care that patients might reasonably expect from it.

In short, lack of confidence in the pharmaceutical industry may partly be the result of the failure of the systems of checks and balances which should be helping it to align its activities to public purpose. If the industry is to have a healthy future – and it is in everyone's interest that it does – it must accept the need for accountability. This is not just because society wants the industry to explain and justify what it does; it is also because the industry positively needs checks and balances on its power. Without this discipline, the industry will always be in danger of losing control of itself and failing as a result.

Professional Drug Information

There are two distinct consumer views of professional drug information. The normative view – one which is probably quite close to the "image" the industry gives of itself – is that *the information about drugs that manufacturers give should fairly reflect all relevant information about the benefits and costs of that product; and positively prompt the physician to use a product as well as he or she possible can.*

On the face of it, this seems a reasonable expectation – and close enough to the "scrupulous regard for truth" that the industry claims to observe [5]. It suggests a standard which, if decently observed, would greatly improve the ways in which drugs were used and also ensure that products competed primarily on their merits. Moreover, it can work.

I have referred elsewhere to the information package provided with the Alza Corporation's *Progestasert* interuterine contraceptive system [6]. This demonstrated to my satisfaction that such standards can work – though I admit that my satisfaction was partly due to the belief that the Alza initiative is probably decades ahead of its time. How many pharmaceutical companies, for example, at present make a point of giving physicians the kind of information that will persuade them to use a better (drug or non-drug) alternative if it is available? And how many companies give physicians enough information to choose realistically between competing products – at the same time withholding information which tends to have the opposite effect?

The reality of the present situation is that professional drug information supplied by the industry accords with commercial rather than scientific norms. By this I mean that there is a gross bias towards providing information about the benefits of drugs and the widespread acceptance of many standards which, in my view, would stand no chance whatever of meeting with public approval [7]. I offer no evidence for this view, not least because it would take a book or more to support it adequately. I state this simply as a deeply held personal conviction, suggesting it as a matter for urgent debate.

Why Are Standards Low?

It might, however, be useful to try to explain some of the main reasons why I think this situation occurs. I suggest the following in no particular order of significance:

1. The state of the art of risk management and assessment is rather as one might expect shortly after the end of a period of several thousand years in which medicine has done more harm to consumers than good [8]. That situation has begun to be reversed, but only in recent decades. The result is that basic technologies and understandings are still unfolding, and that changes (for better and worse) are being made at a considerable speed. We pretend we are on top, perhaps because individually we are blinded, deafened and otherwise overwhelmed by this rate of change. But – assuming we have a future – the fact is we still have nearly everything to learn.
2. We are also, hopefully, at just the very beginning of a new era for human kind – one in which there has at last been some serious consideration of the notion that citizens and consumers have basic needs and rights. But, equally, we have a very long way to go – given for example that most people in the world are positively ill, though the means certainly exist to make most of them quite well.
3. Relatively few of the pharmaceutical industry's products are yet actually unique enough to be promoted for what they are and to survive commercially. The implication is either that we use to get fewer, better products – or that we have to tolerate considerable distortions of the whole truth in drug information and a degree of underhand promotion.
4. We have yet to work out who is responsible for what. As things now stand – although the industry is pre-eminently in a position to take responsibility – it choses to justify its usual practices essentially on the grounds that they appear good enough to government and the medical and allied professions. For the reasons outlined, this is not nearly good enough.

In relation to this last point, it should be emphasised that the "consumer view" is far from being just that. It is not an isolated view – if it were, the consumer movement would have made nothing like the recent headway that it has. It is obvious from its impact that the consumer movement in fact articulates views that are quite widely and increasingly held in government, in the medical profession and elsewhere.

I would accept the criticism that consumer activitists have tended to exaggerate the down-side of drug use. I see this essentially as a response to the industry's reflex tendency to advertise the triumph of benefits over costs – though that is no excuse. This further underlines the need for some meeting of minds.

If Nothing Is Done

What will happen if consumers continue to feel apprehensive either about drug products or about the quality of information which affects the way in which they are used? To generalise sweepingly, I would suggest that they will overwhelmingly benefit (because consumers need to be more cautious about drug use) and that the industry will largely bear the cost.

The main reason for suggesting that the industry stands to lose is that consumers tend to have views about drugs generally, rather than about specific products, simply because they are in no position to discriminate between individual drug products or information packages. Thus, if consumers lose confidence through experience with individual products, they will tend to be much more cautious about using any one. And inevitably they will spread the word.

There is already evidence of considerable and growing disenchantment with drugs generally. Alternative medicine, for example, clearly implies alternatives to drug use. The recent and rapidly-growing trend to demand compensation for drug injury is another manifestation of the same thing. There is also now evidence that consumers are taking prospective action. There are, for example, already clear signs of consumer resistance to the consumption of new drugs – on the grounds that their effects are less well-known and/or less easy to predict than the effects of older drugs. This is obviously threatening to an industry which puts such a high premium on innovation.

The fact that consumers react as they do clearly implies that the whole drug industry may suffer even if it is only a minority of companies that step badly out of line. It follows, unfortunately, that there are limits to what individual companies can do even if they are firmly committed to make progress. Unilateral action may not be enough to succeed.

Where Do We Go from Here?

The first question to ask is whether we – meaning mainly the industry in cooperation with the true consumers of its products – go anywhere. The answer to this question is unclear, even if the consequences of inaction are not. Consumers can be expected to support the pharmaceutical industry only to the extent that the industry does the same for them.

Thankfully, we seem to be moving away from the situation in which the industry has willingly allowed itself to be spoken for by the intellectual counterparts of Rambo. These characters seem to have had little or no clear idea of what it is consumers have been complaining about – and, in my view, have done the industry an enormous disservice by suggesting it was not even worth finding out.

I interpret the occasion of this conference as the beginning of the end of such "philosophies". I very much hope it will emerge as a turning point: and I have no doubt that the organisers wish it to. However, what will happen must depend largely on the participants – and this will take time to be revealed. It should not take too long.

The impression I have from talking to some of the moving spirits behind this conference is that their worst fear is that participants may leave the conference thinking that there is not really much that needs to be done – and/or if there is, that it would not be up to them to do it. I have to say I think this is an unduly pessimistic view. No company with its ear to the ground could consciously decide that this risk would be worth taking.

I would like to think that my worst fears about the outcome of this conference are equally unrealistic and pessimistic. My worst fear is that the participants here will appreciate the enormity of what needs to be done, but will be daunted by the prospect of making the progress which is needed. It is true there is much to be done – but it can be done, with support from the consumer movement, once there is real commitment to do it.

If there is a middle way, I suggest this conference will emerge as one of the clearest signposts to it. In the context of "risk management and assessment", the key to making the progress that is needed is to identify with the people who take risks. They will then indentify with you.

References

1. Medawar C (1987) Failings of the pharmaceutical industry. Pharmaceut Med 2: 259–263
2. World Health Organisation (1983) New approaches to health education in primary health care. Geneva, TRS 690, p 19
3. Braithwaite J (1983) Corporate crime in the pharmaceutical industry. Routledge and Keegan Paul, London
4. Teeling-Smith G (1983) The future for pharmaceuticals: the potential, the pattern and the problems. Office of Health Economics, London
5. International Federation of Pharmaceutical Manufacturers Associations (1981) International Code of Marketing Practice
6. Medawar C (1986) No news, good news? SCRIP 1162, 10 Dec. 1986, p 18
7. Medawar C (1988) Data sheets: a consumer perspective. Lancet I: 777–778
8. Henderson LJ (1935) Physician and patient as a social system. N Engl J Med 212: 819–823
9. Ingelfinger FJ (1977) Health: a matter of statistics or feeling? (editorial) N Engl J Med 296: 448–449

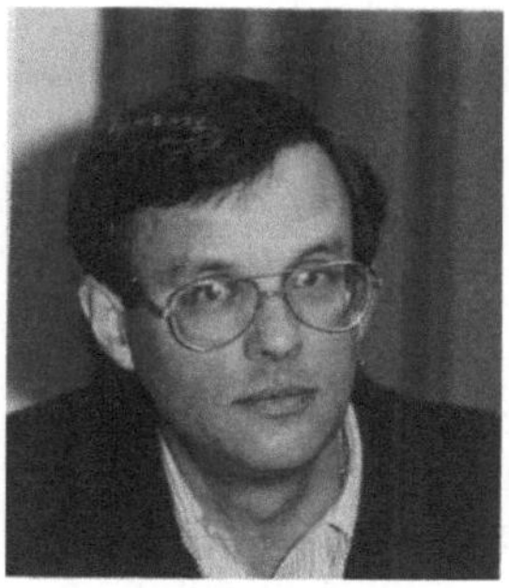

17. Going Patient, Going Public

P. F. Carpenter

The Pharmaceutical Marketplace

Twenty years ago most patients felt comfortable being told what to do by their physicians. In today's society, with much better communication and with the government and media playing far more dynamic roles, patients' needs – met and unmet – can now focus on pharmaceutical products.

The media and others have become increasingly active in scrutinizing the health care system. Stories about unexpected damage to an individual frequently make the front page of newspapers. Consumer advocacy groups have also become much more militant in the areas of health care and pharmaceutical products. Medawar (this volume) has made useful observations about what consumers think and feel and about their expectations of how the pharmaceutical industry should conduct its affairs.

The government is also increasingly concerned with protecting the public from the risks of pharmaceutical products. Ensuring that beneficial products get to market – even when they have a suitable risk-to-benefit ratio – has therefore become of secondary importance. This attitude has evolved because the government is the first to be criticized when a beneficial product is found to have undesirable side effects, even if such effects occur only in a very small group of users or in patients for whom the drug was never intended to be prescribed.

Thus, in the United States and elsewhere, patients' expectations are changing dramatically with respect to standards of care, standards of information, and the quality of health care and pharmaceutical products. Yet even though patients demand more time and information, physicians and pharmacists – because of economic constraints on the health care system – find it increasingly difficult to give them the time they want.

In the United States in particular, all these developments frequently lead people who have great, if not realistic, expectations about pharmaceutical products to seek legal redress if the expectations are not fulfilled. As a result of increases in financial settlements and of court rulings on product liability, the cost of product liability insurance has skyrocketed.

Divergence between expectations and reality is where the industry – and individual companies – have most often gotten into trouble. Drug developers have often told the world that they have the "magic bullet" to cure one of its ills, but consumers argue that these same developers have inadequately conveyed some of the side effects. Better understanding of customers' needs and desires in this area will produce better products [1].

Going Patient, Going Public for Better Communication

Individual pharmaceutical companies – and the pharmaceutical industry as a whole – must now contemplate how to respond to the changing marketplace. One change would be for individual pharmaceutical companies to consider "going patient, going public." This phrase implies at least three types of improvements in communication:

Communicating with the Patient. In those instances where the United States Food and Drug Administration (FDA) requires direct communication from the pharmaceutical manufacturer to the consumer, we must compile clear and appropriate patient information and make it readily available. In addition, we will need innovative ways of communicating the risks and benefits of pharmaceutical products.

Communicating with Physicians. The physician's role as intermediary is crucial, so we should strive to strengthen that role and to provide the physician with the best communication tools possible. This means, among other things, providing more appropriate information on the full spectrum of drug actions.

Improving Patient-Physician Communication. We may be able to stimulate fruitful and relevant communication between physicians and patients. We already spend much time informing physicians about our products. By reaching out to them, and also to pharmacists, with expanded information we can encourage greater mutual trust between physicians and patients. Such mutual trust, as Professor von Wartburg points out (this volume), cannot be bought; it must be earned.

The Benefits and Risks of Informing Patients

The Benefits

We must recognize that the patient is a potentially powerful ally in the pursuit of improved drug therapy. We should not assume that patients are not capable of or interested in taking an active part in any therapeutic intervention or preventive activity. The closer the patient comes to becoming an informed ally of the pharmacist and physician, the more satisfactory the therapeutic outcome is likely to be. Informed patients will know what questions to ask; physicians will better know how to answer them.

Since a well-informed patient is much less likely to misuse a product, the gap between patient expectations and reality will decrease. Informed patients, for example, tend to achieve better compliance with their regimens and thus to receive better therapy. Furthermore, they are more apt to be appropriate patients.

It is shocking to realize that one inappropriate patient's use of a pharmaceutical product has the potential for costing the pharmaceutical company many times the profit from that product's appropriate use. Thus, improved patient targeting and selection are essential in preventing drug disasters. With better informed patients, we are much less likely to receive unpleasant surprises.

The Risks

The risks in better informing patients are significant. Nevertheless, physicians and pharmacists need to take more time to ensure that patients are well informed because in the long run everyone pays a greater penalty for inadequate information. The industry, for example, may spend $ 100 million and many years in bringing a medically superior pharmaceutical product to the marketplace. If it then introduces this product without taking precautions to prevent its misuse, the result may be that a good product is suddenly, and without recourse, removed from sale because it caused significant problems in a few inadequately cautioned patients.

To better inform patients, it is unavoidable that we give visibility to otherwise obscure risks. Greater visibility may create a short-term competitive disadvantage compared with providing less information; that is, incomplete disclosure may create the illusion of greater safety. This illusion, however, cannot be maintained in the long run.

As a result of being better informed, some patients may use fewer drugs or take smaller doses of drugs. On the other hand, with increased compliance, some patients may use larger doses simply because they will more closely adhere to the prescribed regimen. If the patients who discontinue drug use are high-risk individuals, their discontinuance can be a substantial benefit to the pharmaceutical company.

Obstacles to Better Informing Patients

The obstacles to better informing patients are many [2]. The subject matter is complex and therefore difficult to describe in lay terms. Patients' abilities to deal with complex matters vary tremendously, even when communications are carried out at a lay level. Furthermore, some patients simply lack interest in becoming informed about pharmaceutical products.

Regulatory constraints also vary significantly between countries. The United States, for example, is reasonably supportive of efforts to provide more information to patients. Other countries (e.g., the United Kingdom and the Federal Republic of Germany) are unconvinced that fuller disclosure of drug risks and benefits is appropriate for patients, or that it would even work.

Some lawyers' apprehensions center on the belief that each change is fraught with great risk. They feel that, in providing patients with additional information, pharmaceutical companies may jeopardize themselves by implying that previous and current levels of information are inadequate.

Corporate discomfort may also afflict any pharmaceutical company that has basked in the illusion that many of its products are largely without hazards and now is expanding its efforts to communicate its drugs' risks. Such communication is, at least at first, a difficult act, and one that is expensive. Moreover, it usually has not been done previously on a systematic basis.

In view of these obstacles, it seems clear that any company that wants substantially to increase the amount of information that it communicates must develop new expertise and capabilities within its staff.

Pharmaceutical Hardware and Software

Pharmaceutical hardware comprises the actual drug and dosage form. Pharmaceutical software includes the information provided to facilitate the rational use of the hardware – the package, physician package insert or label, patient package insert or label, professional promotional information, and details of aids for physicians and pharmacists.

All this software may be the best "insurance policy" that a pharmaceutical company can buy. The information provided helps physician, pharmacist, and patient cooperate in making an informed choice on using or not using a product on the basis of a comprehensive understanding of its risks and benefits.

Yet within the pharmaceutical industry, innovation in software is largely a remarkably unappreciated activity. The industry should review – and, where indicated, increase – its investment in research and development for software and in the use of this software with its products.

Informed Consent: An Historical Perspective

Informed consent began to emerge as a legal concept when people became concerned about whether individuals had actually consented to medical intervention. Eventually the term evolved to become a medical concept.

The Legal Evolution of Informed Consent

Legal case law is a superb historical tool, providing insight into the history of an important societal issue, as reviewed by Faden and Beauchamp [3a]. They cited, as the earliest legal reference to what we now call informed consent, the case of Slater versus Baker and Stapelton in the United Kingdom in 1767:

> ... and indeed it is reasonable that a patient should be told what is about to be done to him, that he may take courage and put himself in such a situation as to enable him to undergo the operation.

The emphasis here is simply on informing the patient in order to encourage him or her to have surgery. In the 1914 case of Schloendorff versus Society of New York Hospitals [3b], this concept emerged as consent plus choice:

> Every human being of adult years and sound mind has a right to determine what shall be done with his own body; and a surgeon who performs an operation without his patient's consent commits an assault, for which he is liable in damages.

In this case the legal issue of battery was of concern rather than the ethics of the situation or concern for the patient's moral rights.

The Nuremberg Code – the first informed consent code prescribed by an outside tribunal for medicine – was developed in 1947 as a result of the extensive "medical" experiments done by the Third Reich during World War II. This code [3c] defined informed consent as follows:

This means that the person involved should have legal capacity to give consent; should be so situated as to be able to exercise free power of choice ... and should have sufficient knowledge and comprehension of the elements of the subject matter involved as to enable him to make an understanding and enlightened decision.

This code was later confirmed in United States courts. In the 1957 case of Salgo versus Leland Stanford Jr. University Board of Trustees, the landmark decision combined the words "informed" and "consent" for the first time to create the expression "informed consent." The courts ruled that physicians have the duty to disclose "any facts which are necessary to form the basis of an intelligent consent by the patient to proposed treatment" [3d].

Medical Evolution of Informed Consent

Within medicine the evolution of informed consent began with surgical procedures, which were invasive by their very nature. Informed consent was subsequently used for some generally noninvasive medical procedures, then for clinical trials of pharmaceutical products, and finally for some marketed pharmaceutical products.

In 1964 the Declaration of Helsinki [3e] was the first code of informed consent prescribed internally by a professional body in medicine:

In any research on human beings, each potential subject must be adequately informed of the aims, methods, anticipated benefits and potential hazards of the study and the discomfort it may entail [and] that he is at liberty to abstain ... The doctor should then obtain the subject's freely given informed consent.

In the United States, the FDA in 1966 defined informed consent [3f] as follows:

"Consent" or "informed consent" means that the person involved has legal capacity to give consent, is so situated as to be able to exercise free power of choice, and is provided with a fair explanation of all material information concerning the administration of the investigation drug, or his possible use as a control, as to enable him to make an understanding decision as to his willingness to receive said investigational drug.

This definition referred exclusively to clinical trials and not to commercial use of pharmaceutical products.

In the case of Canterbury versus Spence (1972) [3g], the concept of informed consent was further developed:

The context in which the duty of risk-disclosure arises is invariably the occasion for decision as to whether a particular treatment procedure is to be undertaken. To the physician, whose training enables a self-satisfying evaluation, the answer may seem clear, but it is the prerogative of the patient, not the physician, to determine for himself the direction in which his interests seem to lie. To enable the patient to chart his course understandably, some familiarity with the therapeutic alternatives and their hazards becomes essential.

It is useful to reflect on the medical community's reaction to informed consent in the early 1970s and to compare this reaction with the ready acceptance of informed consent a mere 10–15 years later. As Faden and Beauchamp [3h] point out, the medical community's initial response was negative:

Physicians saw the demands of informed consent as impossible to fulfill and – at least in some cases – inconsistent with good patient care. In tone the articles ranged from serious critique to caustic parody. Dire predictions were voiced that fearful patients would refuse needed surgery after disclosure.

In 1973, however, the American Hospital Association [3i] dealt with the issue of informed consent as follows:

The patient has the right to obtain from his physician complete current information concerning his diagnosis, treatment, and prognosis in terms the patient can be reasonably expected to understand ... The patient has the right to receive from his physician information necessary to give informed consent prior to the start of any procedure and/or treatment.... The patient has the right to refuse treatment to the extent permitted by law and to be informed of the medical consequences of his action ... The patient has the right to obtain information as to any relationship of his hospital to other health care and educational institutions insofar as his care is concerned.

Clearly the American Hospital Association was moving toward providing substantially more information, or at least the right to more information, to its patient customers.

By 1982 the concept of informed consent had developed significantly, and Jonsen [3j] was able to provide a particularly clean, concise, and simple definition of it:

...The willing and uncoerced acceptance of a medical intervention by a patient after adequate disclosure by the physician of the nature of the intervention, its risks and benefits, as well as of the alternatives with their risks and benefits.

In 1984 the American Medical Association dealt with informed consent in some detail:

The patient's right of self-decision can be effectively exercised only if the patient possesses enough information to enable an intelligent choice. The patient should make his own determination on treatment. Informed consent is a basic social policy for which exceptions are permitted where the patient is unconscious or otherwise incapable of consenting and harm from failure to treat is imminent; or when risk-disclosure poses such a serious psychological threat of detriment to the patient as to be medically contraindicated. Social policy does not accept the paternalistic view that the physician may remain silent because divulgence might prompt the patient to forego needed therapy. Rational, informed patients should not be expected to act uniformly, even under similar circumstances, in agreeing to or refusing treatment.

Philosophy of Pharmaceutical Informed Consent

The philosophy of pharmaceutical informed consent is based on three presumptions:

- Each individual is the master of his/her own body (the concept of autonomy).
- Each individual has a right to decide whether or not to use a pharmaceutical product (the concept of choice).
- In order to make such a choice, the individual must have adequate information (the concept of being informed).

The physician and pharmacist are essential to making these presumptions work, but they can be effective only if they have the tools needed to perform their role in the best possible manner.

A Proposal

The pharmaceutical industry should adopt a concept of pharmaceutical informed consent – or, perhaps more properly, pharmaceutical informed choice – that reads as follows;

> The patient's right of self-decision can be effectively exercised only if the patient possesses enough information to permit an intelligent choice. Therefore, the physician and pharmacist should have adequate information about a pharmaceutical product and its alternatives so as to assist in the presentation to and understanding by the prospective user. Pharmaceutical product information for patients should be used to inform patients about a product's benefits and risks rather than promote the use of the product.

This concept – the next logical step from the previous concepts of informed consent – will be viewed by many as a radical proposal. My purpose in suggesting this concept is to stimulate the dialogue, not decree the outcome of that dialogue. The concept of pharmaceutical informed consent is not meant to be thought of as a theoretical idea. Instead, it should be regarded as something that has evolved from a very difficult situation, and that has been tested in the marketplace with a specific product.

Progestasert System: A Case Study

In 1986, when the Progestasert system, Alza's intrauterine contraceptive, suddenly became the only IUD remaining on the United States market, we had the opportunity to test our ability and willingness to enlarge the scope of our information to the patient. Acting through the physician, we provided extremely extensive information on this contraceptive.

One company that had marketed an IUD had gone bankrupt, and all other IUDs had previously been removed from the United States marketplace by their respective manufacturers. There clearly were strong reasons for us to consider removing our product from this marketplace. There was also a strong reason to keep it in the marketplace: the Progestasert system was now the only IUD available for women who could not use other methods.

Alza's software innovation began with its very difficult decision to keep the Progestasert system in the United States marketplace. This decision had required extensive consultations with physicians, lawyers, consumers, and critics and the development of a unique patient information leaflet in an informed consent format. This exercise was tremendously valuable to us as a learning experience, and the adversity of the situation provided a tremendous impetus for innovation.

The Progestasert system's new patient package insert is a seven-page document for the physician to give to the patient; it provides extensive information so that the prospective IUD user can know in detail the risks associated with the use of the Progestasert system. The format of the patient information leaflet encourages interaction between the patient and physician by requiring the patient to initial the end of each section. Furthermore, it also includes a list of topics that lets the patient know what she should discuss with her doctor or nurse practitioner. Once the patient has read the entire leaflet, discussed its contents with the physician or nurse practitioner, had all her questions answered, and been advised of the risks and benefits of Progestasert system use, she can make an informed choice on whether or not she will use the product.

There is no attempt in this package insert to sell the product, and every effort is made to prevent its use by inappropriate individuals or against the patient's will. Our 2 years of experience with this informed choice and consent method for the Progestasert system has been superb. The introduction of this document has met with broad support from many sectors of the consumer movement.

Conclusions

We can summarize the points discussed here as follows:

- The patient has the right to make an informed choice on the use of a pharmaceutical product.
- Adequate information about the benefits, risks, and alternatives is a prerequisite for making an informed choice.
- The physician and pharmacist are essential intermediaries in the informed consent process.
- The pharmaceutical industry has the capability of helping the physician and pharmacist achieve informed patient consent.
- The long-term benefits to the patient of informed consent and informed choice far outweigh the risks to the pharmaceutical industry.
- Competition in the quality and value of information should be as vigorous as the competition in the creating and marketing of new chemical entities.
- Any move toward pharmaceutical informed consent – as with any change – will and should involve controversy, debate, and dissension.

References

1. Carpenter PF (1983) Understanding risk. Med Dev Diagnost Indust 5 (6): 24–26
2. Carpenter PF (1987) Responsibility, risk and informed consent. Presented at the National Academy of Engineering, Institute of Medicine, in press
3. Faden RR, Beauchamp TL (1986) A History and Theory of Informed Consent. Oxford University Press, New York

3a :	p 117	3h :	p 91
3b :	p 123	3i :	p 94
3c :	p 282	3j :	p 283
3d :	p 125		
3e :	p 156		
3f :	p 282		
3g :	p 134		

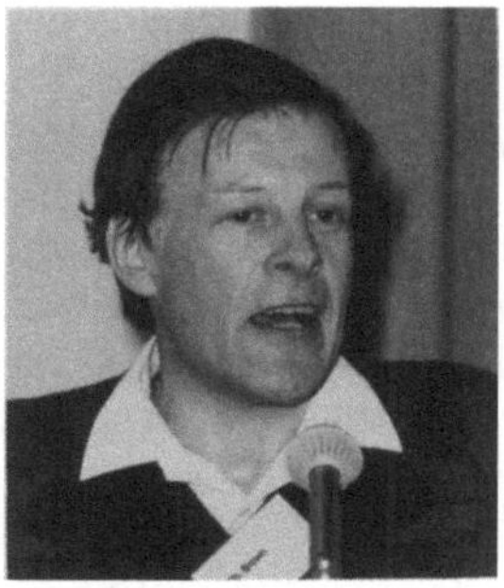

18. Reporting Adverse Drug Reactions: The Media Approach

P. J. Brown

Introduction

Before discussing in detail the relationship between the pharmaceutical industry and the media, I would like to make some general observations about the role of the media.

In ancient times, it was sometimes the practice to kill the messenger who brought the bad news. To a certain extent this still happens today, although blood is not shed. Whenever the news is bad, the first reaction of the recipient is to criticise the media either for getting the information wrong or for presenting a distorted picture of the event. And when the news is continuously bad, the media is accused of being biased.

On the other hand, those who present the news see their task, first and foremost, as presenting a mirror on life and events. If the recipient does not like what he or she sees, reads or hears, then this is, in fact, more of a commentary on what is being reported than a comment on the media itself. I would go further and say that what biases there are in the media have built up over time and are a consequence of the continuous slant that the news has taken year in and year out.

It could also be suggested – flippantly – that if you want to see a better reflection in the media mirror, you should get a face-lift. The more serious answer is that those who make the news should be come more aware of the image which they create. This image depends as much on the things that are not said and not done, the silences and the refusals to comment, as it does on all the fine words that are uttered.

Turning now to the main body of my text for this presentation, I think it is fair to say that pharmaceutical companies would like to find effective ways of reducing media interest in reporting about adverse drug reaction (ADR) problems. This is for a number of reasons. The industry believes that the media (a) distorts ADR issues, exaggerating their severity; (b) takes the view that the company must have been involved in wrong-doing; (c) puts pressure on the regulators and authorities to take hasty and ill-considered action with respect to the drug involved; and (d) unfairly chastises the manufacturer for being mean and heartless in the amount of compensation that it pays to the innocent victims.

One school of thought, not a million miles away from this conference, believes that education is the answer to the media problem. It says: "If only we can get the media to realise that there are risks, as well as benefits, associated with the use of medicines, their interest in the subject will wane, and the problem will diminish or possibly go away."

I believe that this approach fails because it does not recognise why the media are interested in reporting ADRs. It is not simply a matter of editors and journalists failing to understand that risks are associated with drug treatment. If this were true, and since we know in precise numerical terms the risks associated with the various forms of travel, there should be no stories in the press about airliners falling out of the sky, multiple crashes on motorways, ferryboats sinking on the high seas, or high street shoppers being killed by trucks. These are not completely unexpected or previously unknown to happen, but they are news stories.

I would, of course, stress that the remarks that I have just made are in the context of the reporting of drug risks by the media. I am not saying that it is not important to do everything possible to understand, quantify and evaluate risks with new and established medicinal products – which is the main thrust of this conference. What I am saying is that the media are not interested simply in drug risk and do not need to be educated about it.

To change media reporting about ADRs, particularly those which result in products being withdrawn from the market, it is important first to understand why the media – press, television, radio and other communication channels – are interested in the subject.

In the space available here, I would first like to suggest some of the reasons for media interest in reporting about ADRs and discuss some of the key aspects of ADR reporting; second, examine the question of what effects ADR media reports have on the industry; and, third, give some ideas about the things that companies could do to reduce the problem.

Media Reporting of ADRs

The media interest in ADRs must be seen in the context of its interest in medicine. Because of its universal relevance, medicine is of great interest to the media. On the scale of things, it probably comes a close third after politics and sex. Media stories are broadly about progress towards an earth-bound immortality or about quackery in the pursuit of this objective. Stories involving ADRs and their victims are generally classified as being stories about quackery, which basically means false medical claims and exploitation of the sick for profit.

Given this general approach, it is hardly surprising that the starting point for the journalist investigating an ADR story is that innocent people have been harmed when they thought they were being helped; that the provider of the treatment must have been either less than honest in his claims or negligent in the way that he conducted his experiments; and that doctors and authorities were duped or bribed. His task is to prove that any or all of these assumptions are true.

It is important, I believe, that nothing has happened over the past several years of reporting about ADRs to change this basic perception of the problem. The stories are still about innocent victims and guilty manufacturers. You may think that I am exaggerating when I portray the problem in these crude terms, but let me assure you that this is the way in which the media approach the subject.

I have been surprised by the comments of journalists working for the public media. Clearly, they still have a deep distrust of pharmaceutical companies. Inevitably, their knee-jerk reaction to an ADR story is that the company concerned must have been up to the old trick of putting its interest in sales and profits before the interests of the patients, and now it has been caught.

Am I, then, admitting in fact that the media have failed to understand that drugs have risks as well as benefits, and that, therefore, there is still good reason to try to educate them about the inevitability of ADRs in order that they will write more objectively and understandingly in future? Indeed, you may well argue that the only way to overcome the prejudice that I have described is by education, particularly about the basic problem of the risk-to-benefit ratio of medicines.

Whilst it may be the case that the risk-to-benefit argument has not been understood or accepted by the media, I believe that the reason why media attitudes have not changed is that the media are unable to handle drug-related crises in the same way as comparable events in other areas of public interest.

To understand this comment, we should look at the way in which the media approach other "disaster subjects", the category into which ADR reports inevitably fall. Where other disasters are concerned, the media reaction is to find out what went wrong, and what lessons are to be learned. The reader then knows that the risks of a repetition are at least significantly reduced, and the world is a safer place in which to live.

When an airliner crashes, for example, the media set out to report what happened, how it happened and why. They report when the black box has been recovered. They publish photographs of the disaster area, complete with the strewn belongings of the unfortunate passengers, to show the scene. If there are survivors, they are interviewed for the whole world to have first-hand evidence of what happened. After this, there is the report of the public enquiry. Finally, there are the conclusions, the lessons learned, the apportionment of blame, the changes to the systems, the compensation and the punishment, put on record for all to see and read. The same is true when a ship goes down or an industrial plant explodes. So at the end of most disaster stories, it is possible to close the book and say, we know what happened and why, and we are at least better off for knowing.

But is this what happens with ADR disasters? On the basis of what has happened over the past few years, it would seem that the answer is "no". There are two basic problems facing the media and the public that they serve. First, unlike other disaster subjects, there are no set safety criteria for medicines, and, second, it is virtually impossible to undertake a full public examination of what happened and why. This results in far from satisfactory conclusions being reached about causes of ADR disasters – and frustrated media determined eventually to get things out into the open. For the media, the pursuit of the pharmaceutical "bad guys" goes on. They are also intensely distrustful of the "companyspeak" on matters such as risk-to-benefit ratios and the like, which they see as excuses for not coming clean with the facts.

I would like to make the point that we have so far heard in this meeting about ADRs and issues of drug safety. This, however, is not the issue for the media. What interests the media is not the risks of the drugs but discovering who the people are who make the decisions that expose patients to these risks, and not only who the people are, but how they arrive at these decisions. If the who and how were known, the whole problem of drug risks would be better understood, and this could improve the odds against their happening again.

I make this point strongly about the importance of the decision makers for the media, particularly because we all know that there are problems with risk assessment of drugs. The question is how do people make such important decisions about releasing relatively untested drugs on the basis of essentially inadequate safety information? And since this meeting is about risks of drugs, let me remind you how shaky the ground is when we start building castles on drug safety foundations.

First, companies talk a lot about the need for the media to understand that medicines have risks as well as benefits, and that the real issue is the risk-to-benefit ratio seen in the context of the seriousness of the disease being treated. But the media know that the data from which the levels of risk and benefit are calculated are, in fact, assembled by the company itself and not by an independent body, and that the company is far from perfect.

By contrast, in other areas the risks are more clearly established, understood and analysable. With an airliner, for example, there are physical construction criteria that must be met; there are procedures that must be followed for maintenance and flying; and there are rules for pilots, engineers, management and those responsible for the safe passage of the plane through the airways. In the aftermath of a disaster, all these can be publicly examined and assessed.

But is this the case with a pharmaceutical? The risk-to-benefit ratio of an NSAID, or a strong analgesic, or an antibiotic is an imprecise concept, more often than not quantified after the event, and not based on any component parts or readily analysable set of criteria. Risk-to-benefit for medicines may be a fine concept, but it seems to be based on very little hard fact.

And how good are companies at calculating drug risks? They acknowledge that in the period immediately following the introduction of a drug onto the market the level of patient exposure is not sufficiently extensive to allow a full determination of the ADR profile. This can happen only when several million patients have been treated. So how reliable is the risk-to-benefit ratio in the early years of a new drug on the market, when many of the ADR disasters occur?

We have also heard a lot over the past few years about the problem of measuring accurately the incidence of ADRs. Doctors are notoriously bad at recording adverse events and recognising them as ADRs, and even when the industry tries to be more scientific in its post-marketing surveillance efforts, there are still major hurdles to be overcome before reliable statistics can be compiled. The absence of sound mortality and morbidity data makes the identification of some of the rarer and more serious ADRs virtually impossible.

And to confuse matters still further, the question is always in the mind of the investigative journalist: "How honest has the company been with the numbers?" – given the periodic revelations about less than honest researchers in clinical trials.

Overriding all of this, the regulatory authorities do not appear to be particularly effective in policing drug safety. And this does not help public or media confidence. Since they lack the facilities to undertake independent evaluation, the regulators are forced to rely on the scientific and medical evidence presented by the company whose drug they are considering. As we well know, much of this evidence is of a confidential nature so it never sees the light of day. Is it surprising, then, that the national drug watchdogs are regarded as ineffective when they are called on to handle an ADR crisis and they cannot produce the evidence on which they have made their decisions?

In the context of the weaknesses of the basic safety data, can one blame the media for wanting to find out how the marketing decisions were made, and by whom? If one wants an example of the lack of satisfactory public investigations of ADR disasters, one need look no further than the recent case of Lilly and its drug Opren (benoxaprofen). Despite the thousands of words that have appeared in the medical and lay press, what really do we know about the Opren ADR story? Importantly, in the Opren case no national authority had the powers to review publicly what happened, so what information is available is fragmentary and incomplete in a number of key respects. With the company adopting a policy of settling cases out of court, there was little opportunity to have access to the data submitted for registration, which remain confidential.

There has been very little information published in the medical literature about the alleged victims of the various Opren ADRs, so all we have is charge and countercharge about the various ADRs reported. In particular, no scientific or medical light has been thrown on the validity of the claims that some patients suffered from long-term photosensitivity caused by the drug, something which, if true, is a novel phenomenon deserving careful study. Numerous questions remain to be answered, ranging from the appropriateness of Lilly's marketing, the responsibilities of company executives, and the compensation paid to the victims. All these are matters which affect public confidence in the pharmaceutical industry and its member companies. They also contribute to the attitude of the media to the industry.

I am not saying that Lilly is guilty of wrong-doing, other than in the particular instance in which wrong-doing was admitted. But when seen in contrast with other issues of similar public interest, the absence of a full public enquiry is to be regretted. With the Lilly case, as with the many others which went before it, what public lessons have been learned, so that if a similar episode happened again clear charges of negligence could be brought? The answer is none. It has been left to the company to decide behind closed doors what steps, if any, need to be taken. From the point of view of the media and the public, this is not good enough.

Importantly, I would accept that in many cases a full public enquiry would clear a company of blame and dismiss many of the charges brought against it. This in itself is an important aspect of the problem. At present, whilst there are no guilty companies, there are no innocent ones. Hence, the suspicions remain, the system of product evaluation for safety and efficacy is not seen to be modified in order to cope better with the problems underlying the ADR disaster, marketing methods go unchanged, and the critics and the media remain frustrated.

Effects of Media Reporting Upon Industry

Where do we go from here? Perhaps we should look briefly at the effects of the adverse media reporting on the companies whose products have been under the spotlight. As I see it, there are, broadly, two effects at the company level – first, there is the immediate effect on the product under suspicion, and, second, there is the effect on the company itself.

There can be little doubt that intense media attention can lead to the withdrawal of a product either voluntarily or by government order. This effect is now so evident that companies are withdrawing their products even before the media searchlight picks up the problem. Among such firms we find Johnson & Johnson; Farmitalia; Berk/Revlon; Merck, Sharp & Dohme, and Hoechst.

In more scientific terms, the willingness of companies to withdraw new and established products for safety reasons means that they are appraising risks more carefully and acting promptly when there is a significant negative shift. It is interesting to note that risk evaluation has components which go well beyond scientific and medical calculations. This can be exemplified by the withdrawal of Osmosin by Merck, Sharp & Dohme. The serious ADR problem was identified in the United Kingdom, and the product was withdrawn from that market. This resulted in the parent company having to take worldwide action. Importantly, the risk-to-benefit ratio of Osmosin related not only to the product in the context of its competitors, but also to the prescribing environment in the United Kingdom, where there are no original packs or patient package inserts, and where the level of doctor advice to patients is probably amongst the lowest in developed countries.

Since drug withdrawal is virtually a worldwide phenomenon, it is clear that national environmental factors have an important role to play. The effect can also be seen in Ciba-Geigy's withdrawal of its clioquinol product, where Japanese usage patterns resulted in European holiday makers being deprived of an important element in their holiday travel kits.

The second effect is on the company itself. Here, experience of a public ADR problem undoubtedly has an effect on the internal workings of the organisation. But, as I have said, in the absence of public information, we have very little hard and fast evidence to go on. From a business point of view, it is interesting to consider whether companies are harmed by the adverse publicity that they receive at the hands of the media.

Regarding the financial evidence, the conclusion must be that there is little immediate commercial effect other than that arising from the withdrawal of the product. But for a major company relying on a wide range of products for its sales revenues, the loss of a new product does not appear to present too many problems. Importantly, it is seldom, if ever, that the negative effects "spill over" onto the prescribing and sale of other medicines. In fact, there is evidence in some cases of a sympathy reaction, and sales of other preparations increase.

In conclusion, therefore, it seems that the effect of negative media reporting about a company's product is likely to be confined only to the product in question. It may have an effect on the internal workings of a company, but beyond this there is little long-term damage. Perhaps this is why the issue of media relations does not get the attention that some feel that it deserves.

The occasional media storm is seen as being precisely that, a short-term phenomenon which passes, doing little general damage. Perhaps if there were effective boycotts of a company's product, more attention would be paid to the problem.

Improving the Relations Between Media and Industry

So what should companies do about their media relations? Even if they do not think that they have a problem now, they could well have one in the future, given the determined efforts of their critics, who will not go away. Put simply, I believe that they should adopt a two-pronged strategy. First, they should avoid trouble, and, second, they should be better at handling trouble when it happens. Both call for a far greater awareness of what the media challenge comprises.

By way of a backdrop to my closing remarks, I would say that it must be assumed that the media are investigative and independent. Good relations with the media is only another name for a trade-off between the handling of the current news and some other story, present or future. Sympathetic handling by the media is not to be relied on. I say this because there are those who say that it is important for companies to establish good relations with the media in the expectation that such action will result in less critical reporting and better management of the news by the company. That is a false expectation, since it is based on a complete misunderstanding of the work of journalists and those who direct them.

As I said earlier, the task of the journalist is to investigate and report in the expectation that when things have gone wrong someone is to blame. The likelihood of a company being able somehow to manage the news by establishing good relations with relevant journalists is also naive since it ignores the fact that behind the journalist are editors who demand that stories are properly handled. Also, one newspaper or television channel cannot afford to ignore a sensational story which is being carried by all the other media.

Provided a company limits its expectations of the relationship with journalists to hoping that more accurate information is published, then it is a worthwhile exercise to cultivate relations to the media. But in my experience, the hope is always there that the bad news will be suppressed. This culminates in the phone call in which the company's public relations man says: "I'm very disappointed in the way you handled the news about our particular problem. I thought we had built up such a good understanding, and now this has happened."

A second piece of general advice is stay out of fights that have nothing to do with you. Let me explain.

Recently, in the United Kingdom there was a very critical television programme about the use of a Wyeth tranquilliser. Representatives of both the company and the Association of the British Pharmaceutical Industry (ABPI) had been invited but refused to attend, and the problem had to be discussed in their absence. The programme set out to show that the tranquilliser in question caused horrendous withdrawal problems for the unfortunate patients who were prescribed it, and that blame should be laid at the doors of the company for its irresponsible and incomplete marketing which had failed adequately to warn about the hazards of the therapy. In the absence of the company and the ABPI, the debate was forced to concentrate on the decisions of the doctors and the needs of patients, representative groups of each being present along with members of various help groups and promoters of alternative treatments. The result of the debate was to show, first, that the problem had little, if anything, to do with the marketing practices of Wyeth. It was clearly a very complex medical issue, with patients suffering from hard-to-define conditions and with a wide range of medical opinion about how best to administer treatment. This, after all, is the truth, and the implication that the company was going around creating addicts in order to generate sales was nothing more than an obscene suggestion which did nothing to further understanding of what should be done.

Companies must think carefully about whether they want to be involved in the discussion of issues which, if carefully analysed, may be seen to have nothing to do with them. Questions about the proper use of medicines are medical ones and should rightly be discussed by the doctors who prescribe and the patients who take the treatments. The presence of the pharmaceutical company in such debates almost inevitably distracts attention from the central issues.

Too often the pharmaceutical company has considered that it must be present when its product is being discussed. My advice is stay away, tell the media to talk to the doctors who use it and let them explain their actions and reasons.

This last point really leads me to the two main points that I want to make about media relations, the first of which is avoiding trouble. The avoidance of trouble can be translated into the avoidance of risk, and this is really a matter of company culture. Looking back at some of the bad news stories about pharmaceutical companies and their products, one cannot help but conclude that at the bottom of it all there were some poor decisions taken which put the company at risk. Perhaps one can be charitable and say that the problem was not very obvious at the time. But I would ask, for example, whether marketing an old product with an ADR profile far worse than newer products was not a risky enterprise? And was this risk not exacerbated when the products were being actively sold in Third World countries?

If lessons are to be learned from the media handling of ADR stories in recent years, they should surely include far better monitoring of ADRs (which is happening in many companies) and far better control over marketing to avoid claims that can cause trouble; this is not happening to the extent that it should – marketing men seem to be the last to learn.

I was recently involved in a discussion about the desirability of companies having their marketing activities audited by outside organisations. I see considerable problems in getting such a scheme off the ground. However, if one considers the auditor role to be important, I do not see why an internal auditor could not be put in place by an enlightened and determined management to ensure that, at all levels and in all markets, the company's marketing activities meet predetermined standards.

As I said at the outset of this talk, media reports about drug hazards are about patients who have been harmed. But a properly and promptly compensated patient is not news, and a properly informed patient has little about which to complain. So the challenge to the pharmaceutical industry is to take the news appeal out of the situation, that is, remove the disaster element from the situation. This is done by ensuring that the patient is properly informed about his or her therapy and the risks associated with its use, and by ensuring that the doctor and the pharmacist are supplied with appropriate literature, compiled preferably by a medical or consumer body which is independent of the manufacturer.

And whilst I am on the subject of avoidance of trouble, I believe that there should also be some form of independently operated compensation scheme for the victims of unforeseen drug risks. This should be run by government and industry, with compensation in the no-fault situation relating to actual loss, controlled by a ceiling amount and a menu of damages and compensation. Where the patient is harmed because he or she has not been fully informed about a known side effect, the doctor should be sued. Where a manufacturer's negligence is suspected, the issue should be resolved in the courts, with awards taking pain and suffering into consideration and the directors of the company risking criminal prosecution.

Finally, what should a company do if it finds itself in difficulties with the media over the safety of one of its drugs? Obviously, what I have said about compensating patients and taking the heat out of the situation is essential. But having said this, I would stress the need for companies to be prepared for such a situation.

In my experience, companies which have run into difficulties from patients alleging harm by one of their drugs are poorly prepared to deal not only with the media but also with the situation as a whole. Too many companies operate in the pious belief that it cannot happen to them – which shows how little they understand the risk aspect of pharmaceutical product marketing. Every airline tries hard to avoid disaster, but I am sure that they all have a procedure for handling the unthinkable, because the odds are that it will happen one day.

The absence of any operational plan for handling the media in a crisis is one of the major reasons why the press are so persistent. But frankly, one would be horrified at the stupid things that companies do and say when the press phone for information. Senior executives are absent, questions must be sent as telexes, replies take days to be given, "legalspeak" takes over, and the hatches are all battened down. That is not the way to behave – and companies which adopt this posture get the bad press they deserve.

I would end by urging all companies to set up procedures at local market and international levels for dealing with the media in the event of an ADR disaster affecting one of their products. This should involve simulated crisis training. Not only would this approach improve the way in which a company handled the media when one of its drugs was in trouble, but it would also make the company think deeply about the overall policy that it should adopt for handling such matters. A lot of the trouble comes because there has not been adequate thought given to the problem in advance, and the company is, therefore, ignorant about how to behave.

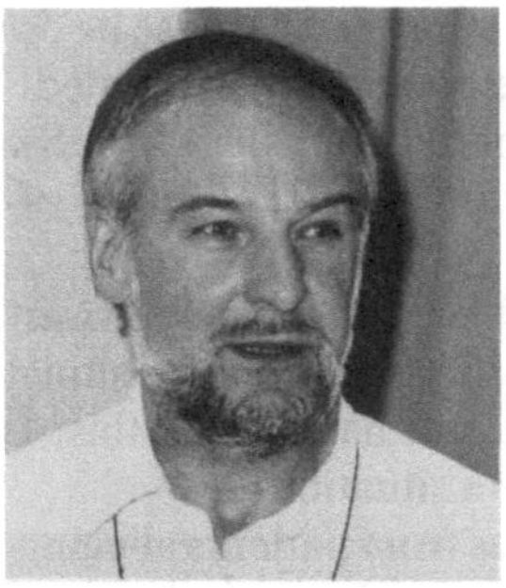

19. What Can Be Learned from Drug Safety Issues?

G. LEWANDOWSKI

Drug safety issues have become a permanent element in the activities of the pharmaceutical business and in public debate on drug therapy. An analysis of the past 25 years, i. e., starting with the Thalidomide disaster in the early 1960s, reveals certain characteristics which merit more careful study when aiming at improving drug safety and reducing the occurrence of safety-related issues.

Lack of safety is the most serious accusation to be raised against a drug. It implies that the drug in question seriously damages the life or the health of patients, and it rapidly makes the issue a public one. This means that equally rapidly a variety of actors and parties with different backgrounds, perspectives, and interests become involved. The actors are the pharmaceutical manufacturer, academia, the medical and other health care professions, regulators and politicians, public interest groups, and the media. These involved parties are not homogeneous and by no means profess homogeneous views. This diversity is one of the reasons why it is so difficult to arrive at generally accepted solutions and to devise equally accepted strategies and procedures for improvement.

This may be a surprise to those who, in line with traditional thinking, believe that drug safety decisions – or, more explicitly, evaluation and decision making on the benefit-risk relationship of drugs – are an exclusive domain of the medical profession, preferably of treating physicians, and that they can be easily derived from clinical trial results and leading manuals, reliably predicted, and if necessary reproduced on the basis of internationally recognized criteria. Reality teaches us a different and more complicated lesson: many more parties, disciplines, principles, criteria, procedures and interests must be integrated into the decision-making process.

There are some other insights that recent history of drug safety issues has to offer. Not all major safety issues that finally led to product withdrawals or severe restrictions of their recommended usage originated as such or were, so to speak, dictated by the properties of the substance, of its unavoidable or uncontrollable adverse effects. In many, if not most, cases, classical and repeated errors lead to the final and fatal verdict on the product and the therapy. In most of these cases it was the manufacturer himself who committed these errors. These include:

- Exaggerated claims
- Heavy promotion with subsequent rapid market penetration
- Unduely high dosage recommendations
- Neglect of particular patient subsets susceptible to more sensitive responses

- Deficient methodological knowledge
- Undue confidentiality of data on efficacy and safety of marketed products
- Undue emphasis on the company's products and clinical studies
- Failure to evaluate data in an international context
- Failure to react speedily and visibly
- Failure to demonstrate human concern and compassion

Efforts at improvement will have to take this into account and give necessary consideration and weight to:
- The substance
- The product information
- The actual usage of the product
- The general conduct of business activities (business ethics)
- General political behavior and communication

Of course, it all starts with professional state-of-the-art evaluation of a given drug during all phases of its life-cycle according to the criteria of quality, efficacy, safety, usefulness, medical need, and cost-effectiveness. This can only be done in a truly interdisciplinary process comprising the following:
- Chemical and pharmaceutical disciplines
- Biological disciplines
- Toxicology and pharmacology
- Clinical medicine in hospitals and in the field including general practitioners
- Clinical pharmacology
- Epidemiology and biostatistics
- Regulatory and economic disciplines

Representatives of each discipline have their word to say; none can boast of an uncontested prerogative, and none can pretend to hold the whole truth. All of them must make decisions based on scientific theories and data but must keep in mind that these are open to controversial interpretation and professional and public dispute. They must make decisions under uncertainty. Here realities and perceptions are closely intertwined, and it is exactly here that value judgments enter, and public interest, concern, and participation are only too legitimate [1].

This is why the manufacturer who is primarily responsible for the safety of his products must organize and successfully conduct:
- An integrated multidisciplinary approach in evaluation, decision, and implementation
- An integrated multidepartmental and international response to safety problems, concerns, and issues
- Transparency of procedures that allow for public participation

On the way to improvement we must successfully pass the milestones of:
- Scientific and technical expertise and competence
- Political sensitivity
- Consequent implementation of professional convictions in the marketplace
- Competent, candid, and credible communication

We could start with cooperation and harmonization in collecting data, with permanent exchange of data on efficacy and safety of marketed drugs, with candid and public discussion of controversial facts, interpretations, evaluations, and issues. It would only be a beginning, and rapid progress and improvement are necessary.

Reference

1. Hutt PB (1978) Unresolved issues in the conflict between individual freedom and government control of food safety. Food Drug Cosmetic Law Journal 33: 588–589

20. Summary of Part III: Presentations and Discussions

The pharmaceutical industry should realize that consumers are bound to question increasingly what it does. Because of the impact that pharmaceuticals can have upon the public at large and because of past problems with drugs, consumers feel that they cannot rely on government and/or the medical profession to question the pharmaceutical industry. The industry will have to convince consumers that it is responsive to the needs of the people who take risks in order to also obtain the benefits of drugs.

The evolution of the patient from a passive recipient of pharmaceutical products to an active consumer must be recognized and accepted by the industry. The very nature of pharmaceuticals is being challenged, and this has given rise to the use of "informed consent" of the patient using a drug. Here, the patient decides whether to use a drug, based on information provided to him by his physician, pharmacist, and the manufacturer of the drug. The marketed drug itself, therefore, must be accompanied by carefully researched information which includes both the benefits and the risks of the product. This must be more than merely packaging or promotion of the drug. In order to build a relationship of mutual trust and respect with the patient, innovation, courage, compassion, committment, and diligence are needed. Competition in the quality and value of the information that the pharmaceutical company provides to the consumer is an important new challenge for the industry. The move toward phar-

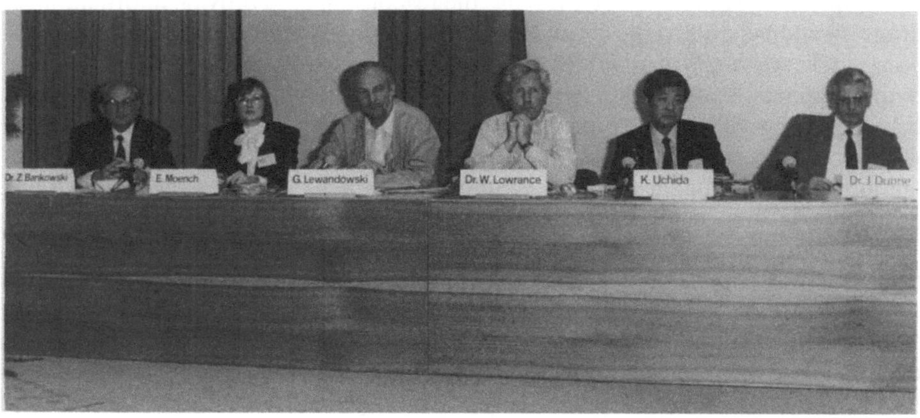

maceutical informed consent, however, will involve controversy, debate, and dissension.

A look at media coverage of drug safety issues shows that reports about drug hazards are, in fact, about harmed patients. If the pharmaceutical industry believes that the media distort adverse drug reaction issues, it should remember that the media behave like a mirror, reflecting what is happening, including what is sometimes a distorted situation. It should also remember that a properly informed patient has little to complain about, and that it is the pharmaceutical company's responsibility to ensure that the patient is properly informed about the therapy and the risks associated with drug use. It is the doctor's responsibility to inform the patient about risks and precautions when prescribing a drug. The mere fact that the media – or the patient – know about the risks, however, does not mean that the risks will be ignored by the media when a problem develops. With any drug problem, the media expect immediate first-hand information about the incident, to know who was responsible, and what can be done about it.

Some advice to pharmaceutical companies was offered by a member of the media: do not try to seduce the media, do not fight other company's fights, and learn to avoid trouble. If a company has a new drug on the market which is better than an older similar drug, it should remove the inferior drug.

Media interest lies with the patient's concerns. The pharmaceutical company should learn to show compassion for the patient. Finally, pharmaceutical companies should be better prepared for drug problems, should have crisis-management training programs, and should, by all means, be able to respond quickly to both media reports and requests for information.

It was observed that, where there are individual victims, real or imaginary, and particularly where there are many of these, and where compensation has been generously given in other countries, it is absolutely impossible for a drug company to win in a case of alleged adverse drug affects. Even if a pharmaceutical company wins in the courts, it still must explain why there are people who allege that they are victims. It is in the pharmaceutical company's own interest to look urgently for those who might be adversely affected by a drug and prevent them and others from being hurt by a company product. Companies which act with this foresight will be at a fantastic competitive advantage.

The question was raised as to who has the responsibility to provide information on drug risk and benefits to the consumer. Is it the drug manufacturer or the physician? Some studies have shown that 75% of physicians do not provide adequate information to their patients. Other questions must also be asked: Should information on risks and benefits be provided before or after a prescription is written? How can one tell whether the consumer is an avid information seeker, someone who only wants a short description of the medication, or is among those who do not want to make any decision regarding medication?

The patient should certainly be informed and consulted about risks and benefits of a drug before any prescription is written, because this is the decisive and often the dismissive act on the part of the prescriber.

It is surprising that more pressure by patients and consumer groups is not put on doctors to provide better information about prescribed drugs. Much medical failure may be attributed to doctor failure; patients fail to get either the right information or the right prescription. The patient should be considered as more intelligent than some studies show him to be.

There was general agreement that the pharmaceutical industry should move toward a policy of the patient's informed consent. It was pointed out that the philosophy of individual autonomy lies behind informed consent, and neither the pharmaceutical company, the physician, the pharmacist, nor the health care organization will be able to deny this autonomy if the consumers want it. Although there is the possibility of providing information that consumers do not want, they should at least have the opportunity to turn down that information. The physician must be the intermediary, the person who presents and explains the product information and the medical information, and who discusses the consequences in relation to the patient's condition. If the industry cannot find ways to provide information to the physicians and ensure that they use it more adequately and consistently, the industry is in trouble.

The idea of a patient package insert was commended, but questions about its practicality and use were raised. There have been legal concerns about patient package inserts as well as concerns from pharmacists and physicians. There are also considerable difficulties in creating an insert, given the differences in education and languages of patients using the products. While the idea of the patient package insert is not without problems, it is a step in the right direction.

Further comments reflected that not only industry is considering patient package inserts, but the European Community is considering them, the Council of Europe has already made recommendations for them, and the Association of the British Pharmaceutical Industry has issued a proposal setting up guidelines for information which should be included in them. What remains is to decide exactly what should be communicated, how, and for whom.

The question of patient information is a complicated issue and should be carefully researched. One may find one reaction from patients when they are approached with a theoretical set of questions and another reaction when they are sick, and specific questions are asked. There is also tremendous variability in what people want to have in the way of information. Some do not want to have choices or to make decisions; others, however, are just the opposite. Information overload is also a problem; so much information on a drug may be provided that patients may actually miss something as important as the possibility of death from taking the drug. Information is not synonymous with tranquility. A patient may say the risk of a drug outweighs the benefits but take the medication anyway because he feels his physician probably knows more than he does. Another problem, at least in the United States, is that physicians are not paid for taking time to talk with patients, and discussion of risks, benefits, and options is time consuming.

Participants suggested that there should be flexibility in providing patient information, and different kinds of approaches should be found for different kinds of patients. Some speakers said that they think patient package inserts would not be prepared best either by the government or the industry but rather by health professionals with sound scientific information.

One panel member maintained that an important reason for freedom of information is that the decision maker will know that his decision may be examined, and that he may have to justify it. Ultimately, the reason for patient information, he said, is to remind those responsible for the regulation, manufacture, and the prescribing of drugs that the purpose of their activity is to help the patient.

It was suggested that the pharmaceutical industry needs some sort of central compensation scheme for patients who suffer from unknown adverse drug reactions. Several participants pointed out that such an effort should incorporate compassion into the compensation scheme; the emphasis, in fact, should be not on the financial side but on the side of compassion for the patient.

Several discussants supported the idea of moving away from a system which is dominated by litigation and large damage settlements against pharmaceutical companies. One pointed out that in the United States, such a system is encouraged by lawyers who get 40% of damages. There are precedents such as no-fault auto insurance and workmen's compensation. A move in the pharmaceutical industry should be in the direction of making settlements fairly and promptly and avoiding the excesses of the legal system. However, one member of the panel cautioned that if compensation becomes the responsibility of the industry, it could become a screen for bad prescribing. There are currently compensation schemes in several countries which have already moved in this direction. But it is important to consider some questions in regard to these schemes: these include: (a) what are the expectations of compensation? and (b) when do people become eligible for compensation?

Compassion should also be considered, but it would be better to consider it separately. If a patient suffers from a well-known adverse drug reaction and should have been warned, is the patient entitled to compensation? The responsibility is on the doctor to warn the patient, and if this is overlooked, the responsibility and problems fall upon the industry. No-fault liability still includes the provision that the patient must prove that he was harmed, and that his was a new and unforeseen reaction. The patient is not covered if the adverse drug reaction was forewarned. And, of course, negligence by either companies or doctors will remain a matter for the courts to decide.

Part IV

Responding to the Issues

21. Editor's Note

Responding to the issues involved a wide array of project reports and proposals that were first presented in four working groups and later discussed in a general meeting. The contributions from the floor helped clarify the issues and contained a series of valuable suggestions. These have been incorporated into the descriptions of the individual projects. Participants agreed that cooperative studies at the international level are necessary.

In this part of the book the reader will find a description of the specific project proposals in a standardized format. Workshops focused on the four main topics that were presented in the course of the conference. These are briefly characterized below.

Pharmacoepidemiology

The sharing of existing data bases and other resources was recommended as a first step for the pharmaceutical industry. The systematic building up of a broad international data base will permit improved and earlier understanding of signals from the reporting system and will aid in the prevention of product attacks and withdrawals. The compatibility of languages and terminologies, however, is an important presumption. The essential prerequisites of such a data base are (a) quality of data, (b) credibility of the organizations in charge, and (c) continuous evaluation and speedy reporting.

In light of these needs, the different types of possible organizations (industry-sponsored or independent) have advantages and disadvantages. Case-studies and the education of industry management, physicians, government, and others are candidates for additional projects.

Risk Perception Analysis

Risk perception by the public, the media, the authorities, and physicians must be ascertained on a regular basis. There is a lack of reliable data. Reports from Sweden and Japan clearly illustrate the gap in knowledge, showing some surprising results, on the one hand, and indicating the need for more open questions, on the other. The surveys done in the two countries should be considered as a start in the collection of data on risk perception. Future work might include international evaluations and applications. The extent to which public perception (and even behavior) can be influenced has been demonstrated in areas such as smoking, alcohol consumption, and driving without seatbelts. Changes are possible but require the investment of time and money. Very often the media are confronted with a need to deliver a quick statement based on available information, when a more comprehensive report would be desirable but cannot be accomplished within a short time.

Communicating the Benefit/Risk Relationship

The role of the media is very important in risk communication. This role comprises mainly three parts: (a) putting an issue into the public eye, (b) setting the agenda of discussion, and (c) influencing perceptions.

A critical problem in communication is the input of information. This is a field in which further improvement is needed, particularly in the pharmaceutical industry. Mistakes in the quantity and quality of information released to the media have damaged the image of the industry. A permanent dialogue between the media and the industry should be initiated.

Risk Appraisal on an International Scale

Improved risk appraisal involves the interpretation of data with more transparency and the setting of priorities to make risk-related decisions easier. Risk appraisal should not be based solely on a system of comparisons of pharmacoepidemiological data but should also refer to other sources of information (e. g., data on the benefits of a drug, the needs of physicians, patients, and authorities, and patient and liability situations). Improved risk appraisal can protect marketed drugs as well as those in development.

22. Pharmacoepidemiology

Comparative Data Base Analysis

Background. A number of well-known data sources are used for pharmacoepidemiological studies. Many of these have limitations. There are additional data sources (those developed for managed care plans, group practices, and hospital inpatient and outpatient care) which have not yet been studied but might offer more complete data than the traditional sources.

Objectives. The purpose of this project is to prepare a comprehensive review of available data sources for drug benefit/risk assessment.

Proposed Activities. An exhaustive survey of available data sources for drug benefit/risk assessment will be conducted. An inventory with all data elements delineated will be developed. A descriptive handbook for use by researchers in selecting appropriate sources of information will be prepared. The handbook will include an international catalogue of data bases on the following items:

- Drugs and diagnoses in general populations (outpatients and inpatients)
- Diagnosis-specific data bases
- Drug-specific data bases
- Spontaneous ADR reporting
- Special registries: diagnoses
- Special registries: drugs
- Population drug data bases

Project activities will include:

1. The review of existing literature, reports, data, and comprehensive data systems.
2. Interviews with international experts who are concerned with drug risk assessment and relevant data collection activities.
3. Analysis of findings and preparation of a descriptive report of the data and data collection systems.

As a first step of the project, a review on data bases in the United States, United Kingdom, and Canada has recently been conducted and published. In its current form (see Chap. 30) it represents a structure for a comprehensive approach. It is recommended that further volumes be expanded to include data bases in Europe and the Far East.

Expected Benefits. The final product of this work will be a comprehensive inventory of drug data sources under one cover. This will include a description of data elements and population sizes and a review of the applicability of these data sources to benefit/risk assessment. The guide will be useful for planning future benefit/risk assessment research and for selecting research data sources.

NSAID Data Base

Background. Although nonsteroidal anti-inflammatory agents (NSAIDs) are widely used, it has been difficult to integrate into a complete picture the benefits and risks associated with their use. Most data bases do not cover entire populations, and studies with single-population data bases are usually insufficient. A full understanding of NSAID effects will require the study of their use in several subpopulations. This project could examine NSAID effects in a comprehensive way using multiple data bases for verification of the effects under study.

Objectives. The purpose of this project is to organize a comprehensive international collaborative study of the beneficial and the adverse effects of NSAIDs over a 3- to 5-year period. The study could serve as a model for other comprehensive international benefit/risk assessment investigations. Methods for cost-effective monitoring of beneficial and adverse effects will be explored.

Proposed Activities. Comprehensive data on specific benefits and risks of NSAID products and NSAIDs as a class will be collected. First, data sources will be identified and evaluated, and a model study design will be prepared. Data collection will then begin in the United States and United Kingdom, to be followed by Canada, West Germany, Japan, Sweden, Italy, and France. A system for continuous monitoring of selected effects will be designed and tested during the study period. Plans include cross-comparison of available data bases and the establishment of an international committee of selected experts.

Expected Benefits. This project will provide comprehensive information on beneficial effects and risks associated with the use of NSAID products among various populations worldwide. It will also result in implementation of programs for systematic monitoring of NSAID benefits and adverse effects, and provide an example for the development of improved systems for benefit and risk data collection for other pharmaceuticals.

Management Training in Epidemiology

Objectives. The purpose of this project is to develop educational programs for scientific and administrative managers in the pharmaceutical industry in drug evaluation and pharmacoepidemiology. The objective of short courses and degree programs is to provide key company personnel with the framework required to validate and evaluate scientific data on drugs. This will lead to improved communication both internally and with external agencies including government and the media.

Proposed Activities. This project addresses a need for additional manpower resources in the fields of drug evaluation and pharmacoepidemiology. The program will offer several courses of study including:

1. Management Development Seminars in Drug Evaluation and Pharmacoepidemiology. These are a series of continuing education seminars for senior management. An original pilot project has been planned for Ciba-Geigy. The seminar will be a 9-day intensive immersion program covering subjects such as: fundamentals of clinical science and epidemiology, biostatistics, introduction to risk assessment, principles of pharmacology and pharmacoepidemiology, etc. Following successful completion of the course, a "certificate of attendance" will be issued.
2. On-Site Seminars for Pharmaceutical Companies. These will be prepared in consultation with interested companies. Faculty will travel to the company and offer lectures, tutorials, and problem-solving workshops designed to meet the specific needs of the company.
3. Issues in Managing Adverse Event Reports. This is a series of seminars and workshops which will provide pharmaceutical company personnel with the framework required to validate and evaluate scientific data on drugs.
4. Annual Summer Program in Epidemiology and Biostatistics.

Expected Benefits. This project will encourage the development of needed professional and scientific pharmacoepidemiological manpower resources for industry and government.

23. Risk Perception Analysis

Public Perception

Background. Drug risks should be viewed in the context of other risks. Recently developed methodology has the power to explain public concerns and to predict reactions to events.

The survey instrument contains questions pertaining to the following general categories:

1. Perceptions of risk (images, attitudes, quantitative scales)
2. Perceptions of benefit
3. Evaluations of a prototypical drug risk controversy (acceptability of risk)
4. Trust in various persons and agencies responsible for drug safety
5. Attributions of causality for adverse effects
6. Perceptions of disease states

Objectives. Research should examine perceptions of hazardous activities and technologies and put risks of different natures into perspective. There are a number of target groups which could be looked at in addition to the general public. Data should be collected in a way that permits international comparisons to be made and changes in risk perception to be monitored over time.

Proposed Activities. Surveys of perceived risk should be conducted, using representative national samples in Canada, West Germany, Japan, Sweden, the United Kingdom, and the United States. The survey instrument is designed to:

- Describe public perception of the risks and benefits associated with various prescription drugs.
- Place perceptions of prescription drug risks within a broader context.
- Allow comparisons to be made across populations from different countries and within national samples.
- Provide baseline data that will allow the impact of new drug problems and controversies to be evaluated and allow trends in relevant attitudes and perceptions to be monitored over time.
- Contribute to basic knowledge and understanding of the influence of public perceptions on the sociopolitical environment in which pharmaceutical companies operate.

A survey of this kind has already been conducted in Sweden (see the paper by Slovic et al., Chap. 11, this volume).

Expected Benefits. This research will elucidate public perceptions about the benefits and risks of prescription drugs. The information that is collected will help companies to communicate more effectively about their products.

Physician and Patient Perception

Objectives. The purpose of these activities is to examine the similarities and differences between physician and patient perceptions of pharmaceuticals and ADRs in selected countries.

Proposed Activities. Survey sample sizes of 1000–2000 persons would be used to investigate the following questions:
- To what extent do physicians explain possible ADRs to patients?
- Do patients comply with physicians' orders regarding medicine dosage and schedule?
- How important do physicians and the public think drug information is?
- What are physician and public perceptions of ADRs?
- Who do physicians and the public hold responsible for ADRs and drug risks?

Surveys of physician and public perceptions of pharmaceuticals and ADRs have been completed in Japan (see the paper by Fujino, Chap. 12, this volume). It is proposed that additional risk perception research be conducted in other countries to allow for understanding of perceptions in these countries as well as cross-cultural comparisons of perceptions.

Expected Benefits. This research allows a better understanding of the differences and similarities between different target group perceptions. The research can be used as an instrument of education and consensus building for governments, the media and public-interest groups.

24. Communicating the Benefit/Risk Relationship

Communication Proposals

Background. Effective communication is the result of a four – stage process: listening, understanding, formulating a message, and communicating. The pharmaceutical industry currently implements the last two of these stages while paying little attention to the first two. An industry-wide program on drug safety risk management and perception offers a unique opportunity for pharmaceutical manufacturers to step back from parochial issues regarding specific products and to move forward by promoting understanding and candor on all matters relating to the benefits and risks of drugs.

Objectives. To promote understanding and candor between all parties interested in drugs, thereby improving communication and knowledge.

Proposed Activities. A multidisciplinary steering committee of internationally renowned representatives – from the areas of epidemiology, health economy, sociology, communications, consumer advocacy, medical journalism, and the pharmaceutical industry – should be established to set specific project goals and priorities and to design and implement activities. Suggested activities include the implementation and promotion of:

- An induction program for pharmaceutical company employees, trainee journalists, consumer groups, legislators, and the medical profession.
- Multidisciplinary focus groups involving industry representatives, legislators, consumer representatives, and specialists.
- Debates on medicine with leading experts, industry representatives, the World Health Organization, leading journalists, and consumer group representatives as participants.
- Medical updates on specific disease areas, concentrating on the epidemiology of the disease, prognosis, and outcome of drug intervention.
- Patient group meetings on different topics, with participation from leading experts, industry representatives, and consumer and patient group representatives.
- A general practitioner newspaper on the assessment of drug benefits and risks, communicating benefit and risk information to patients, and the benefits and risks associated with treatment in specific disease areas.

Expected Benefits. This project could result in short-term improvements in knowledge of motivational factors which would, in the long term, lead to easier and more effective communication for the industry.

Participating in the Public Debate: The United Kingdom as an Example

Background. In the United Kingdom patients are ill informed about the risks of medicinal therapy, and their general attitude towards risks is largely governed by media coverage. With the prescribing of medicines, explanations vary from nil to relatively detailed. It is only recently that calls for fuller explanations about the risks and benefits of medicines have been made by consumer and other organizations.

At a meeting with consumers and special interest groups approximately 2 years ago at the Pharmaceutical Society of Great Britain, under the auspices of the Medico-Pharmaceutical Forum, it became clear that consumers would like to have much more information about the medicines they take, including their benefits and risks. The Association of the British Pharmaceutical Industry and the government now support including patient package inserts with medicines, and this move will gradually be implemented. The demand for more information about treatment options and the benefits and risks of medicines is still growing.

Patients should be encouraged to ask more questions about treatment options and their associated benefits and risks. With a better understanding of the options, patients can participate in decision making and thus make the taking of medicine less involuntary and safer.

Objectives. The purpose of the project is the creation of a risk communication center in the United Kingdom to establish and maintain contact with specialists in risk assessment and to engage in educational activities for patients and the public.

Proposed Activities. This project includes plans for:
- Establishment of a collaborative working group of representatives of selected pharmaceutical companies of subsidiaries in the United Kingdom to plan risk communication efforts.
- Creation of a consultant/advisory panel of experts in pharmacoepidemiology, clinical medicine, health economics, and regulatory medicine.
- Organization of scientific symposia, when appropriate, to promote knowledge and facilitate exchange of research data.
- Establishment of communication with patient and consumer groups to promote understanding of benefit/risk issues.
- Communication with a wider public through press articles and by press coverage of public meetings.
- Establishment of a literature and information base for the use of both scientific and public groups concerned about medical risk issues.
- Participation in research related to risk perception, assessment, decision making, and management.
- Integration of the program with risk-related activities in other countries, as appropriate.

Expected Benefits. Improved information on the benefits and risks of medicines could result in an increase in drug safety and improved cooperation between all parties concerned.

Political Intelligence System

Background. Drug issues have their own life-cycles. These usually start with questions and early signals within the company where the drug has originated. Concerns are then voiced in scientific/medical circles. Such concerns usually find their way into the professional press, which is interested in all aspects of drug benefit/risk issues. Once such reports have surfaced, they raise the interest of consumers, patient organizations, and the lay media. They then have a tendency to become political, leading to demands for action by either legislators or drug regulatory authorities. Hearings and administrative decisions may result if preventive action is not taken.

Objectives. The purpose of the proposed activities is to allow early detection of drug issues reported in important professional publications.

Proposed Activities. Sci-Mate/POLIS is a computerized political intelligence and monitoring system of drug issues covered in the professional press. The POLIS data bank screens important professional journals regularly for emerging drug issues. It provides an overview of all drug issues, thus allowing a comparative analysis and evaluation of important trends.

Sci-Mate/POLIS runs on any IBM-compatible personal computer with five quarter diskettes or three half diskettes. Updated diskettes will be available three times a year to subscribers. The data bank will be expanded over time. POLIS currently includes approximately 600 listings. The information is organized with the following template structure:

- Trademark, generic name of criticized product
- Manufacturer
- Therapeutic class, IMS classification
- Short description of event reported
- Summary explanation of cause of criticism, related to either: quality, efficacy, information, cost-effectiveness, or safety issues
- Country of criticism
- Key critics
- Source of reference

Expected Benefits. The POLIS data base allows one to monitor drug issues, and it alerts one to drug issues before they become politicized.

25. Risk Appraisal on an International Scale

Council for International Organizations of Medical Sciences

Background. A major concern for drug regulators, academic epidemiologists, and members of the pharmaceutical industry seems to be the development of a generally accepted approach to the assessment of drug-associated risks in the postmarketing phase in order to achieve safety standards that are both objective and rigorous.

It is necessary that we develop better use of the entirety of biological information about a drug as a means of better protecting and understanding its clinical performance. This biological information can be used to best advantage only if it is channeled into an appropriate international information network and is available for comparative purposes. There is a corresponding need for greater transparency in the way that adverse reaction reports are generated, collated, and analyzed. In addition, more systematic application of existing methods of postmarketing surveillance need to be considered. This transparency needs to extend to the decision-making process in order to provide the basis for more informed public understanding of the scientific, political, and ethical issues involved.

Progress in addressing these issues is likely to occur only if a mechanism is developed to bring opinion leaders from each of the interested constituencies together under the auspices of an accredited and respected scientific organization. The Council for International Organizations of Medical Sciences (CIOMS) has been acknowledged by regulators, academics, and industry as an appropriate body to provide a forum for discussion. CIOMS has established itself as an independent, impartial, and effective scientific organization.

Objectives. Emphasis will be placed on building consensus for a plan of action to improve the management of drug safety risks by pharmaceutical companies, university scientists, regulatory authorities, physicians, and patients. Discussion will focus on the identification of areas in which improvements can be made and the development of recommendations for uniform international standards (e. g., integration of clinical trial and postmarketing data, standardization of ADR reporting, and evaluation of guidelines for releasing ADR data).

Proposed Activities. This proposal outlines activities which span four phases over the next 3 years:

Phase 1. Establish the CIOMS working group (including academic experts, regulatory authorities, and representatives from industry, the World Health Organization, and other concerned groups) to survey the current situation, prepare preliminary recommendations, propose a detailed CIOMS program, and organize a first high-level policy meeting of experts, regulatory officials, consumers, and industry leaders.

Phase 2. Conduct an international consensus conference, cosponsored by CIOMS and the World Health Organization; publish report and recommendations.

Phase 3. Establish expert committees in critical areas to develop options; publish reports from the expert committees.

Phase 4. Submit recommendations to the World Health Organization on the role that it can play in encouraging adoption of state-of-the-art risk management procedures for pharmaceuticals; develop mechanism for the implementation of conference recommendations.

Expected Benefits. The achievement of drug safety standards that are developed as a consensus among regulators, academics, consumer representatives, and industry.

Pharmaceutical Risk Management Activities in Japan

Background. Japan is the second largest pharmaceutical market in the world. Optimal management of drug risks, in-depth understanding of public attitudes toward medicines, and effective communication with the public about pharmaceutical benefits and risks are thus vital for the industry, physicians, and regulatory authorities.

Objectives. The purpose of this project is to encourage collaboration between the Japanese pharmaceutical industry, experts, and regulatory authorities in:
- Applying state-of-the-art data collection and risk assessment techniques for medicines.
- Improving understanding of public perception of pharmaceuticals.
- Developing more effective communication of drug risk and benefit information.
- Developing international standards for drug risk management.
- Planning a long-term agenda for strengthening the management of drug risks.

Proposed Activities. To achieve the project objectives, survey research must be conducted, opinion leaders and decision makers may be consulted as advisors, expert committee meetings may be held, and research and analysis results may be disseminated to concerned groups.

Expected Benefits. This project would result in strengthened risk assessment and decision making for the industry and enhanced benefit and risk communication with the public in Japan.

Establishment of Risk Institutes

Background. Risk institutes have been established by various industries – primarily the chemical, utility, and food industries – to conduct analyses and convene forums on a variety of environmental and health issues. Such institutes render substantial public service in the study of food safety and electric power generation. International pharmaceutical companies have common concerns about drug risk assessment, management, and communication. A center to advance knowledge and skills in these areas could be of great benefit to all interested parties.

Objectives. This project has three objectives:

1. To provide training in drug risk measurement and communication for health professionals in the United States and abroad.
2. To contribute to the refinement of methodology used to assess the benefits and risks of drugs.
3. To focus public attention on the many issues involved in the measurement and communication of drug benefits and risks.

Proposed Activities. This project involves the establishment of a risk center at Johns Hopkins University with an interdisciplinary program for analysis of the benefits and risks of drugs.

A graduate program for masters or doctoral students will build on already existing masters and doctoral level training programs in epidemiology and in health policy and management. A 1–2 year training program for visiting scholars from abroad is also proposed.

Benefit and risk assessment methods will be developed and applied by a team consisting of pharmacoepidemiologists, statisticians, clinical pharmacologists, health economists, psychologists, health policy analysts, and ethicists.

Staff from the Johns Hopkins Center will participate in national and international conferences, symposia, and scientific meetings. They will also organize international conferences at the University.

Expected Benefits. The Johns Hopkins Center for Analysis of the Benefits and Risks of Drugs will provide expertise on the many issues involved in the measurement and communication of drug benefits and risks. The center will contribute to advancing the science of drug risk evaluation. The center will also provide training for health industry professionals in risk evaluation, managment, and communication.

Part V

Outlook

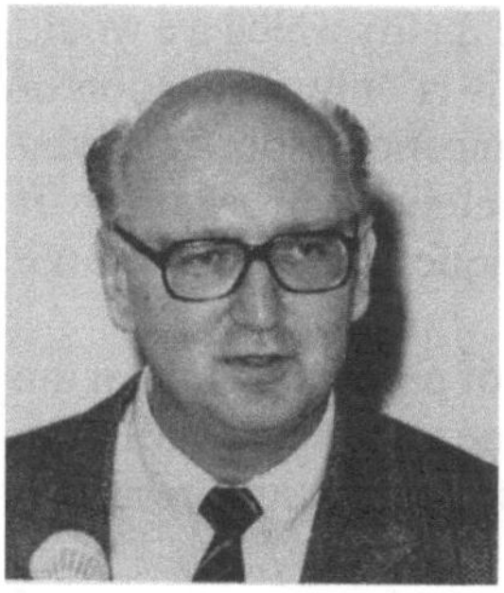

26. The Wolfsberg Questions

W. P. von Wartburg

Instead of making a long-winded conclusion, I would like merely to make a list of questions that have arisen during the course of our proceedings and try to arrange them according to various headings. I have made a number of drafts and circulated them to various people for comments and additions. These questions, the "Wolfsberg Questions," are now grouped together under the headings of risk analysis, risk perception, risk communication, benefit/risk appraisal, and risk management.

I do not propose to go into these questions in detail. Many of them have been raised over the past few days. It is usually the case that more questions are raised than can be answered, but at least one can concentrate on the important points, take them home, think about them, and at some point in time, perhaps one can research certain of the questions.

In addition, I would like to share with you some of my thoughts. I have been asking myself again, why are we having this meeting? Why the concern about drug safety? As I said at the beginning of the meeting, it is our impression that drug safety no longer remains limited, if it ever was, to company-specific issues. Of course, drug safety ranks high among company-specific problems because one must ensure that all the expertise within our companies is available and that competence is demonstrated. But the substance of the problem goes beyond this. We concede that in the premarketing phase, it is more company-specific because it is here that one has all the knowledge. But once the product is in the marketplace, it may become more of a structural issue. In other words, drug safety is at one and the same time a company-specific and a structural issue.

I have also thought again about how one could tackle this issue, and how drug safety, to some extent, has become almost like a cube with 64 sides. Some people consider this to be merely a question of ADR reporting: that if we do ADR reporting in the best possible way, we will know in advance and can react. Yet this is not the whole story, as we may have come to realize over the past 3 days. Some people, on the other hand, say that it is a question of toxicology, or of biostatistics. Some say that it is just a question of clinical studies, that if we do these in the best possible way and have sufficiently large patient populations, we will become aware of all the risks early enough. I think, however, that this is also not the whole story. Nor is it enough to say that if we merely do everything in the phase IV studies or in classical postmarketing surveillance studies, we can evaluate drug safety properly. This is not the whole story either. It is also not just a question of sensationalist media reporting or whatever kind of reporting we may dislike because we feel that this is not the reality which we would have liked to have seen in the media. I do not think that it is only a question of communication; we have focused particularly on the communication aspect, but you can only communicate what you know, and you cannot communicate away a risk. It would be wrong to think that improved communication techniques alone could be the solution to any kind of drug issue.

It is also not only a question of perception. It *is* a question of perception and at the same time a question of value judgements. We therefore need to integrate these various disciplines and approaches in a way which will yield the best possible results in terms of good science and good behavior.

Can any one company do this on its own? Maybe there are such companies, but I have the definite feeling that this is a gargantuan task and that we would be well advised somehow to join forces in certain areas. For example, we have said that we must endeavor to know the maximum possible about our drugs and how they behave in the marketplace. Inevitably, this leads us to the discipline of pharmacoepidemiology. But assessments and judgements surely cannot be made in isolation; we need to examine relative as well as absolute values in order to make valid comparisons. Thus, we need not only pharmacoepidemiology, but *comparative* pharmacoepidemiology. And here there is certainly room for cooperation.

I would like to repeat that this meeting was not a fund-raising exercise. During the past 3 days we took a kind of overall perspective, then concentrated on some specific issues, did more in-depth analysis, and now we have submitted some initial ideas for possible collaborative activities.

I would also like briefly to come back to the meaning of RAD-AR: Risk Assessment of Drugs – Analysis and Response. I think the assessment was here to some extent; the analysis was certainly here, and some of the responses came out as well. Now, I can say with certainty that we will continue with this RAD-AR program, whatever kind of meaning one gives it. We know that we will be traveling down a difficult road and that we will have some setbacks, but we will perhaps have some benefits to show for it. It is my personal conviction that sometimes "getting there" is almost as important as "being there." And I think that if we do the right things and show a willingness to get there, namely to have a better safety and protection element built into our drugs, this is important and will be acknowledged by the world outside.

If I refer to the world outside, I would at the same time point out that RAD-AR is not a Ciba-Geigy public relations exercise. This should be quite clear. We wanted to open up, we wanted to let you know what we are doing, but we did not want to do it in order to make ourselves look good. I also told the media representatives that they were here in order to see what was happening, not to praise Ciba-Geigy.

We at Ciba-Geigy do not think that we know better, nor do we think that we know best. What we want to do is to progress, to go in the right direction, and hopefully have some other companies join in this effort, thereby achieving more than might be possible just on our own.

Three things about this meeting have been rather special, at least for me. First, the fact that you have come – you, who are all direct competitors. In spite of disagreements that we may have in the marketplace, maybe we will find some agreement in the area of protection of public health and assurance of drug safety. Second, what I think is also rather special is the geographical distribution. Sometimes one tends to have meetings just among Americans or just among Europeans. This time we were quite fortunate to have people from all over the world, and I am particularly grateful that our Japanese colleagues have flown here to attend this meeting. The third point that I feel is quite remarkable is the openness on your side: you have come up with suggestions, you have come up with criticism, you have not listened passively but participated actively in all discussions. I hope this openness will lead to a continued exchange on many of these issues. In the context of openness, I want to praise the meeting for having the media and Charles Medawar present. I would like to thank them especially because they have really brought the public, or the consumers, into our meeting.

I must add something else. I felt that sometimes there were defensive tones or defensive attitudes being struck – defensive in the sense that I almost had the feeling that you felt that this was all being done in order to defend our existing or future products. This would be the wrong message with which to leave you. This would, again, be only reactive, in the sense that we would wait until something happened, then defend in the best possible way against whatever we did not want to occur. The idea behind the meeting and behind our plea for collaboration and cooperation is really to improve the state of the art of all our activities, to show competence in what we are doing, to demonstrate it also to the outside world, and thereby, hopefully, to gain, maintain, or regain public acceptance in our respective countries.

It is obvious that good drugs mean good business. But in the end, the goal is to reach out in a better way to the patient, to protect him in an optimal way. You can open any management textbook and read about staying close to your customers, listening to your customers, taking your customers' views into consideration, etc. I feel that for too long our customers have been seen as being only those in the medical profession, and that we have forgotten that there is an endcustomer who really takes our drugs. It is in this context that I think we should reach out to the patient. RAD-AR will hopefully benefit Ciba-Geigy; it will hopefully benefit the industry as well, but, above all, it should benefit the patient. Thank you very much.

Part VI

Annex

27. Curriculum Vitae of Authors

BROWN, PHILIP J., Ph. D.
Publisher and Managing Director, *SCRIP World Pharmaceutical News,* Richmond, Surrey, UK
B. Pharm., London University, UK
Ph. D. Organic Chemistry, Cambridge University, UK
Member of the Pharmaceutical Society of Great Britain; Publisher of *Clinica-World Medical Device News, Animal Pharm, Pharmaprojects, Agrow – World Agrochemical News and Haznews"*

CARPENTER, PETER F.
Chairman of the Strategic Planning Committee, Alza Corporation, Palo Alto, California, USA
1962 A.B., Chemistry, Harvard University, USA
1965 M.B.A. University of Chicago, USA
Chairman of the Board of Directors and Chairman of the Executive Committee, American Foundation for AIDS Research

FÜLGRAFF, GEORGES M., Prof. Dr. med.
Scientific Counselor and member of several committees in the European Community and FRG
Studies in Law, Economy, Psychology and Medicine
1959 M.D., University of Munich, FRG
1972 Professor of Pharmacology and Toxicology, University of Frankfurt/Main, FRG
1974 President of the Federal Health Office (BGA), Berlin
1980 State-Secretary of the Federal Ministry of Youth, Family Affairs and Health, Bonn, FRG

FUJINO, SHIRO, Prof., Ph. D.
Professor, Faculty of Economics, Chuo University, Tokyo, Japan
Ph. D., Graduate School of Hitotsubashi University, Japan

GUESS, HARRY A., M.D., Ph.D.
Senior Director of Epidemiology, Merck, Sharp & Dohme Research Labs., West Point, PA, USA
1972 Ph.D., Mathematics, Stanford University, USA
1979 M.D., University of Miami, USA
Postdoctoral training in Biostatistics and Population Genetics at the National Institute of Health, USA, and in Pediatrics at the University of North Carolina, USA

KRAUER, ALEX, Dr. rer. pol.
President, Chairman of the Board and Managing Director, Ciba-Geigy Ltd., Basle, Switzerland
Studies in Economics at the University of Basle, Paris and the London School of Economics, graduating Dr. rer. pol. from Basle University, Switzerland

LASAGNA, LOUIS, Prof., M.D.
Dean, Sackler School of Graduate Biomedical Sciences; Academic Dean of the Medical School; Professor of Psychiatry (Clinical Pharmacology); Professor of Pharmacology; Director, Center for the Study of Drug Development; Tufts University, Boston, MA, USA
1943 B.S., Rutgers University, USA
1947 M.D., College of Physicians and Surgeons, Columbia University, USA
President, Medicine in the Public Interest; member of Board of Trustees, International Life Sciences Institute; Vice-Chairman, Drug Science Foundation; member of the editorial board of numerous scientific journals

LETZEL, HEINZ, Dr. med.
President, Staticon Gesellschaft für medizinische Forschungsberatung mbH, FRG
1970–1976 Studies in Medicine, Philosophy and German Literature
1976–1979 Postgraduate training in Biostatistics and Epidemiology, Institut für medizinische Informationsverarbeitung, Statistik und Biomathematik, University of Munich, FRG
Lecturer in Biostatistics and Epidemiology, University of Munich, FRG

LEWANDOWSKI, GUENTER
Head of Pharma Policy Department, Pharmaceutical Division, Ciba-Geigy Ltd., Basle, Switzerland
Studies in Law (West Berlin, FRG, and Lausanne, Switzerland); former Vice-President of the Federal Health Office (BGA), FRG

LOWRANCE, WILLIAM W., Ph.D.
Senior Fellow and Director, Life Sciences and Public Policy Program, The Rockefeller University, New York, NY, USA
1965 A.B., Chemistry and Biology, University of North Carolina, Chapel Hill, USA

1970 Ph. D., Organic and Biological Chemistry, Rockefeller University, USA
Member of the Executive Committee of the Science Advisory Board to the United States Environmental Protection Agency; extensive research on risk issues, ethical dilemmas in science and technology, and related policy

MEDAWAR, CHARLES
Director, Social Audit Ltd., London, UK
1965 Graduated in Russian language and literature, Indiana University, USA
Founded Social Audit Ltd. and Public Interest Research Centre Ltd. in 1971. Co-founded Health Action International; in 1985, appointed Scientific Coordinator to a consortium of lawyers acting for 1500 Opren plaintiffs

NELKIN, DOROTHY, Prof., Ph. D.
Visiting Professor, Department of Sociology, New York University, NY, USA
1954 A. B., Philosophy, Cornell University, NY, USA
1977 Professor, Department of Sociology, Cornell University, NY, USA

ORSINGER, JEAN A.
Head of Pharmaceutical Division, Ciba-Geigy Ltd., Basle, Switzerland
Studies in Commerce, Zurich, Switzerland

SACHS, ROGER, M. D.
Vice President, Regulatory Affairs and Clinical Safety, Pfizer Pharmaceuticals, New York, NY, USA
1964 A. B., Biochemical Sciences, Princeton University, USA
1968 M. D., State University of New York, Downstate Medical Center, Brooklyn, NY, USA
1977 J. D. Fordham University School of Law, USA

SLOVIC, PAUL, Prof., Ph. D.
President, Decision Research, Eugene, Oregon, USA; Professor, Department of Psychology, University of Oregon, USA
1959 B. A., Psychology, Stanford University, USA
1962 M. A., Psychology, University of Michigan, USA
1964 Ph. D. Psychology, University of Michigan, USA
Member, Board of Scientific Directors, Risk Sciences Institute of the International Life Sciences Institute; member, Advisory Board, *Journal of Risk and Uncertainty;* member, Editorial Boards, *Risk Analysis* and *Risk Abstracts*

SPITZER, WALTER O., Prof., M. D.
Professor and Chairman, Department of Epidemiology and Biostatistics, Strathcona Professor of Preventive Medicine, Professor of Medicine, McGill University, Montreal, Canada
1962 M. D., University of Toronto, Canada
1966 M. H. A., University of Michigan, USA
1970 M. P. H., Epidemiology and Public Health, Yale University, USA
Editor of *Journal of Chronic Diseases* and founder of *Clinical and Investigative Medicine*

VON WARTBURG, WALTER P., Prof. Dr. jur.

Member of the Pharma Management Committee, Ciba-Geigy Ltd., Basle, Switzerland

1963 Doctorate, Faculty of Law, Basle University, Switzerland

1965–1966 Legal and economic studies at Princeton University and Harvard Law School, Master of Law degree

Professor of Public Health Policy at the Graduate School of Economics, Business and Public Administration, St. Gallen, Switzerland

28. Bibliography

General Risk Topics

Anonymous (1987) Acceptable degrees of therapeutic risks. Scrip 24 June: 22
Aronow WS et al. (1987) Risk factors for atherothrombotic brain infarction in persons over 62 years of age in a long-term health care facility. Am Geriatr Soc 35: 1–3
Bajgier SM (1982) An interactive model of attitude and risk-benefit formation regarding social issues. Policy Sci 14: 257–278
Berando FM (1986) Survivor education: the role of habits, attitudes and risk taking. Death Stud 10: 391–409
Blomquist G (1986) A utility maximization model of driver traffic safety behavior. Accid Anal Prev 18: 371–375
Brauers WK (1986) Essay review article: risk, uncertainty and risk analysis. Long Range Plan 19: 139–143
Breyer F, Fuchs VR (1982) Risk attitudes in health: an exploratory study. National Bureau of Economic Research, Working Paper 857
British Medical Association Guide (1987) Living with risk. Wiley, Chichester
Bühlmann H, Loeffel H, Nievergelt E (1969) Einführung in die Theorie und Praxis der Entscheidung bei Unsicherheit. 2nd edn Springer, Berlin Heidelberg New York
Carpenter PF (1982) Risk assessment. Meeting on risk assessment, National Academy of Science, 10 Feb
Chelemer MJ (1987) The hazardous substances initiative: working to create safer tomorrow. MIT Report May: 4–7
Covello VT (1987) Decision analysis and risk management decision making: issues and methods. Risk Anal 7: 131–139
Covello VT, et al. (1982) Risk analysis, philosophy and the social and behavioral sciences. Risk Anal 2: 53–58
Covello VT, Mumpower J (1985) Risk analysis and risk management: an historical perspective. Risk Anal 5: 103–120
European Community (1980) Nuclear and non-nuclear risk – an exercise in comparability. Final Report, EUR 6417 EN. Pollution Prevention (Consultants), Crawley, UK
Fischhoff B, Lichtenstein S, Slovic P et al. (1981) Acceptable risk. Cambridge University Press
Fritzsche AF (1986) Wie sicher leben wir? Risikobeurteilung und Bewältigung in unserer Gesellschaft. TÜV Rheinland, Cologne
Goodman J (1986) On criteria of insignificant difference between two risks. Risk Anal 6: 235–244
Haight FA (1986) Risk, especially risk of traffic accident. Accid Anal Prev 18: 359–366
Hanley JW (1981) Monsanto's early warning system. Harvard Bus Rev Nov/Dec: 107–122
Helal B (1984) Physical risks in modern sport. Med Sci Law 24: 247–248
Hollaender A (1986) Acceptance of the distinguished contribution award of the society for risk analysis. Risk Anal 6: 113–115
Imhof AE (1981) Die gewonnenen Jahre. Von der Zunahme unserer Lebensspanne seit dreihundert Jahren oder von der Notwendigkeit einer neuen Einstellung zu Leben und Sterben. Beck, Munich

Johnson BB, Covello VT (eds) (1987) The social and cultural construction of risk: essays on risk selection and perception. Reidel, Boston
Kuhlmann A (1981) Einführung in die Sicherheitswissenschaft. Vieweg, TÜV Rheinland, Cologne
Kunreuther H et al. (1984) A decision-process perspective on risk and policy analysis. Manage Sci 30: 475–485
Lave LB (1987) Health and safety risk analysis. Science 236: 291–295
Lowrance WW (1976) Of acceptable risk. Kaufmann, California
Lowrance WW (1986) The ethics of access to health care. Bridge 16: 14–18
Lund AK et al. (1986) Perceived risks and driving behavior. Accid Anal Prev 18: 367–370
Meadows D (1972) Die Grenzen des Wachstums. Bericht des "Club of Rome" zur Lage der Menschheit. Deutsche Verlags-Anstalt, Stuttgart
Medawar C (1986) No news, good news? Scrip 1162: 18–19
Medawar C (1987) Failings of the pharmaceutical industry. Pharmaceut Med 2: 259–263
Miller SA (1984) Introductory remarks to session on risk assessment and risk management. Fundam Appl Toxicol 4: 380–382
National Research Council (1982) Risk and decision making: perspectives and research. National Academy Press, Washington D.C.
National Research Council (1983) Risk assessment in the federal government: managing the process. National Academy Press, Washington D.C.
Nelkin D (1987) The culture of science journalism. Society Sept–Oct: 18–25
Orleans M, Haverkamp AD (1987) Are there health risks in using risking systems? The case of perinatal risk assessment. Health Policy 7: 297–307
Peets JI et al. (1987) The assessment of major hazards: the density and other characteristics of the exposed population around a hazard source. J Hazard Mater 14: 337–363
Rosen S (1981) Valuing health risk. AEA Papers Proc: 241–245
Rothschild L (1987) Risk. Listener 30 Nov
Royal Society Study Group (1983) Risk assessment. Royal Society, London
Ruckelhaus WD (1983) Science, risk and public policy. Science 221: 1026–1028
Ruckelhaus WD (1984) Risk in a free society. Vital Speeches Day 1: 354–358
Schneider T (1981) Grundgedanken und Methodik moderner Sicherheitsplanung. Sicherheitsingenieur 8: 26–30/9: 18–29
Starr C et al. (1980) Risks of risk decisions. Science 208: 1114–1119
Swedish Drug Information Council (1987) The elderly and medicines. Swedish Drug Information Council, Stockholm
Teeling-Smith G (1983) Measuring the social benefits of medicine. Office of Health Economics, London
Tenner E (1987) Warning: nature may be hazardous to your health. Harvard Magazine Sept–Oct: 34–38
von Winterfeldt D, Edwards W (1984) Patterns of conflict about risky technologies. Risk Anal 4: 555–568
Wilde GJS (1987) Theorie der Risikokompensation der Unfallverursachung und praktische Folgerungen für die Unfallverhütung. Unfallheilkunde 130: 134–156
Wilson R, Crouch EAC (1987) Risk assessment and comparisons: an introduction. Science 236: 267–270
Wittmann W (1982) Risikobewältigung: Gratwanderung zwischen Sicherheit und Freiheit. Informationstagung der SVA. In: Neue Zürcher Zeitung, Zeitfragen: 289 (11/12 Dec 1982)
Wynne B (1983) Technologie, Risiko und Partizipation: zum gesellschaftlichen Umgang mit Unsicherheit. In: Conrad J (ed) Gesellschaft, Technik und Risikopolitik. Springer, Berlin Heidelberg New York
Yadigaroglu G, Chakraborty S (eds) (1985) Risikountersuchungen als Entscheidungsinstrument. TÜV Rheinland, Cologne
Young FE (1987) Risk assessment: the convergence of science and the law. Regul Toxicol Pharmacol 7: 179–184

Risk Perception

Batelle-Institut (1981) Untersuchungen über die technischen, organisatorischen und gesellschaftlichen Voraussetzungen für Risikostrategien im Bereich technologischer Entwicklung (Endbericht) RS I/2-510321, SR 70. Batelle, Frankfurt
Borman SA (1983) Origin of risk assessment. Anal Chem 55: 1438a–1440a
Brown J (1987) Risk perception: expert opinion versus public understanding. ESRC Newslett 59: 17–19
Carpenter PF (1983) Understanding risk. Med Device Diagn Industry 5 (6): 24–26
Drabek TE (1986) Human system response to disaster: an inventory of sociological findings. Springer, New York Berlin Heidelberg
Fishburn PC (1984) Foundations of risk measurement. Manage Sci 30: 396–406
Gafni A et al. (1984) Risk attitude and time preference in health. Manage Sci 30: 440–451
Heilmann K, Urquhart J (1983) Keine Angst vor der Angst. Risiko – Element unseres Lebens und Motor des Fortschritts. Kindler, Munich
Jung CG (1975) Über die Psychologie des Unbewußten. Fischer, Frankfurt/M.
Kishchuk NA (1987) Causes and correlates of risk perception. Risk Abstr 4: 1–4
Kletz TA (1983) The mathematics of risk. Interdisciplinary Sci Rev 8:114–119
Kuhlmann A (1978) Sicherheit als Wert in Technik und Gesellschaft. In: Ropohl G et al. Maßstäbe der Technikbewertung. Vorträge und Diskussionen, VDI Tagung, 18 and 19 Nov 1977. VDI Prints, Düsseldorf
Lave LB, Menkes J (1985) Managing risk: a joint US-German perspective. Risk Anal 5: 11–23
Lee TR (1981) The public perception of risk and the question of irrationality. Proc R Soc Lond 376a: 5–16
Lerch I (1980) Risk and fear. New Sci Jan: 8–11
Lowrance WW (1983) The agenda for risk decision making. Environment 25 (10): 4–8
Lowrance WW (1985) Modern science and human values. Oxford University Press, New York
O'Donnell M (1986) The media and their influence on public attitudes to drug development and use. Br J Clin Pharmacol 22: 101s–102s
Otway H, Thomas K (1982) Reflections on risk perception and policy. Risk Anal 2: 69–82
Pochin EE (1975) The acceptance of risk. Br Med Bull 31: 184–189
Schneider SL, Lopes LL (1986) Reflection in preferences under risk: who and when may suggest why. J Exp Psychol 12: 535–548
Slovic P (1987) Perception of risk. Science 236: 286–290
Slovic P et al. (1984) Modeling the societal impact of fatal accidents. Manage Sci 30: 464–474
Slovic P et al. (1987) Risk perception and risk regulation. Administrative Conference of the U.S., Washington D.C., 5 March
Starr C (1985) Risk management, assessment, and acceptability. Risk Anal 5: 97–102
Starr C et al. (1984) A perspective on health and safety risk analysis. Manage Sci 30: 452–463
von Wartburg WP (1984) Drugs and the perception of risk. Swiss Pharma 6 (11a): 21–23
Wildavsky A (1984) Die Suche nach einer fehlerlosen Risikominderungsstrategie. In: Lange S (ed) Ermittlung und Bewertung industrieller Risiken. Springer, Berlin Heidelberg New York

Risk Communication

Anonymus (1987) NRC launches study on risk communication. Risk Newslett June: 13–14
Brushwood DB, Simonsmeier LM (1986) Drug information for patients – duties of the manufacturer, pharmacist, physician and hospital. J Leg Med 7: 279–340
Davies JC, Covello VT, Allen FW (eds) (1987) Risk communication. Conservation Foundation, Washington D.C.
Kasperson RE (1986) Six propositions on public participation and their relevance for risk communication. Risk Anal 6: 275–281
Keeney RL, von Winterfeldt D (1986) Improving risk communication. Risk Anal 6: 417–424
Röglin HC (1984) Kommunikationsrisiken der Großtechnologien. In: Lange S (ed) Ermittlung und Bewertung industrieller Risiken. Springer, Berlin Heidelberg New York

Shapiro S (1985) The decision to publish ethical dilemmas. J Chron Dis 38: 365–372
Sharlin HI (1986) EDB: a case study in communicating risk. Risk Anal 6: 61–68

Regulation

Albert RE (1985) Risk assessment in regulatory decision-making in the EPA. In: Homburger (ed) Safety evaluation and regulation of chemicals 2. Karger, Basel, pp 146–149
Beauchamp TL (1978) The regulation of hazards and hazardous behaviors. Health Educ Monogr 6: 242–257
Bogen KT (1983) Quantitative risk-benefit analysis in regulatory decision-making. J Health Politics Policy Law 8: 120–140
Carpenter PF (1987) Medical device regulation and product liability: responsibility, risk and informed consent. NAE/IOM Symposium, 9 March, in press
Huber P (1985) Safety and the second best: the hazards of public risk management in the courts. Columbia Law Rev 85: 277–337
Mattison N (1984) Regulatory scene. Pharmaceut Med 1: 13–16
Montesano R, Tomatis L (1977) Legislation concerning chemical carcinogens in several industrialized countries. Cancer Res 37: 310–316
Petak WJ, Atkisson AA (1982) Natural hazard risk assessment and public policy. Springer, New York Berlin Heidelberg
Pfund P (1982) Recht und Risiko. Tagung 22–23 Nov, Zürich-Oerlikon, Referat 12. Schweiz. Vereinigung für Atomenergie, Bern
Roth DH, Wyzga RE, Hammerstrom T (1984) The use of risk assessment in developing health-based regulations. ASTM Spec Techn Publ 845: 46–65
Scheuplein RJ (1987) Risk assessment and food safety: a scientist's and regulator's view. Food Drug Cosm Law J 42: 237–250
Schroeder CH (1986) Rights against risks. Columbia Law Rev 86: 495–562
Silverglade BA (1983) The risks of risk assessment and risk-benefit analysis. Food Drug Cosm Law J 38: 318–324
Smith MV (1984) Use of risk assessment in regulatory decision-making. Food Technol Oct: 114–118
Taylor MR (1984) The role of law in risk management. Fundam Appl Toxicol 4: 408–417
Travis CC, Richter SA et al. (1987) Risk and regulation. Chem Tech Aug: 478–483
van Andel FG (1985) On regulating perceived risk. Effective Health Care 2: 231–237

Industrial Risks

Anonymous (1986) Accidents will happen. Economist 10 May: 13–14
Anonymous (1987) Unkalkulierbares Risiko. Wirtschaftswoche 13 March: 36–62
Baxter PJ (1986) From Flyxborough to Bhopal: is legislation enough? Br J Industr Med 43: 1–3
Bohnenblust H (1985) Die Anwendung eines risikoorientierten Sicherheitsmodells zur Beurteilung der Neubaustreckentunnel der Deutschen Bundesbahn. In: Yadigaroglu G, Chakraborty S (eds) Risikountersuchungen als Entscheidungsinstrument. TÜV Rheinland, Cologne, pp 431–361
Hartwig S (ed) (1983) Grosse, technische Gefahrenpotentiale, Risikoanalysen und Sicherheitsfragen. Springer, Berlin Heidelberg New York
Kates RW, Kasperson JX (1983) Comparative risk analysis of technological hazards. Proc Natl Acad Sci USA Nov: 7027–7038
Lagedec P (1982) Major technological risk: an assessment of industrial disasters. Pergamon, New York
Lange S (ed) (1984) Ermittlung und Bewertung industrieller Risiken. Springer, Berlin Heidelberg New York
Moolenaar RJ (1986) The industrial role in risk assessment. Sci Total Environ 51: 75–80
Schön G (1982) Grundlagen der Erfassung und Bewertung technischer Risiken. In: VDE/VDI-Tagung: Risiko – Schnittstelle zwischen Recht und Technik. VDE, Berlin, pp 45–62

Sellner D (1982) Die Bewertung technischer Risiken bei der Rechtsanwendung. In: VDE/VDI-Tagung: Risiko – Schnittstelle zwischen Recht und Technik. VDE, Berlin, pp 183–203
Zerna W (1983) Grundlagen der gegenwärtigen Sicherheitspraxis in der Bautechnik. In: Hartwig S (ed) Grosse technische Gefahrenpotentiale, Risikoanalysen und Sicherheitsfragen. Springer, Berlin Heidelberg New York

Nuclear Risks

Dumenil G (1977) Energie nucleaire et opinion publique. Report 2. ADISH/IREP, Paris, Grenoble
Fritz-Niggli H (1983) Problematik von Risikoschätzungen – Beispiel kleine Strahlendosen. Referat an der SVA/OeAF Informationstagung: Sicherheits- und Risikodenken im Zeitalter der Kernenergie, Zürich-Oerlikon, 22–23 Nov 1982. In: Neue Zürcher Zeitung, Beilage Forschung und Technik 75, 30 March
Fritz-Niggli H (1983) Gefahren der Radioaktivität. Neue Zürcher Zeitung, Zeitfragen: 24, 30 (29/30 Jan, 5/6 Feb)
Fritzsche AF, de Haller G, Nahm W (1982) Die Sicherheit der nuklearen Energieerzeugung: Berichte der SNG zur Kernenergie, Bd 5. SNG, Bern
GRS (1979) Deutsche Risikostudie Kernkraftwerke. Eine Untersuchung zu dem durch Störfälle in Kernkraftwerken verursachten Risiko, Hauptband. TÜV Rheinland, Cologne
Nowotny H (1979) Kernenergie: Gefahr oder Notwendigkeit. Suhrkamp, Frankfurt
Okrent D (1987) The safety goals of the U.S. Nuclear Regulatory Commission. Science 236: 296–300
Société Française de Radioprotection (1977) Colloque sur les implications psycho-sociologiques du développement de l'industrie nucléaire, 13–15 Jan, Paris
Wallace MD, Crissey BL, Sennott LI (1986) Accidental war: risk assessment. J Peace Res 23: 9–27

Environmental Risks

Anderson HA (1985) Evolution of environmental epidemiologic risk assessment. Environ Health Perspectives 62: 389–392
Baird BNR (1986) Tolerance for environmental health risks: the influence of knowledge, benefits, voluntariness, and environmental attitudes. Risk Anal 6: 425–435
Conrad J (1986) Nitrates in ground and drinking water: analysis of policies and regulations. Sci Total Environ 51: 209–225
Daetwyler JJ (1978) Das Erdbebenrisiko in der Schweiz, neue Erdbebenrisikokarten für die Schweiz fertiggestellt. Neue Zürcher Zeitung, Beilage Nr. 175: Forschung und Technik, 14 June
Eichler W (1982) Gift in unserer Nahrung. Die Brisanz der Umweltgifte in Nahrungsketten. Kilda, Greven
Environmental Protection Agency (1986) EPA to publish guidelines for risk assessment. Environ News 25 Aug
Froines JR et al. (1986) Occupational health surveillance: a means to identify work-related risks. Am J Public Health 76: 1089–1096
Hattis D, Kennedy D (1986) Assessing risks from health hazards: an imperfect science. Technol Rev May/June: 60–71
Hotz A (1981) Risiko im Sport und anderswo. Neue Zürcher Zeitung 14 Feb: 37
Lynn FM (1986) The interplay of science and values in assessing and regulating environmental risks. Sci Technol Hum Values 11: 40–50
Ricci PF, Molton LS (1981) Risk and benefit in environmental law. Science 241: 1096–1100
Russell M (1986) Learning to manage risk: Res Manage July: 12–16
Russell M, Gruber M (1987) Risk assessment in environmental policy-making. Science 236: 286–290
Schnitter N (1976) Statistische Sicherheit der Talsperren. Wasser, Energie, Luft – eau, énergie, air 68: 126–129

Chemical Risks

Anonymous (1987) Groundwater. Ciba-Geigy Corp, Toms River, New Jersey
Anonymous (1987) The management of risk. Lancet 4 July: 54
Blokker EF (1983) Erfahrungen bei der Durchführung von Risikoanalysen für einige Anlagen der petrochemischen Industrie in Rijnmond. In: Hartwig S (ed) Große technische Gefahrenpotentiale, Risikoanalysen und Sicherheitsfragen. Springer, Berlin Heidelberg New York, pp 161–170
Drummond MF (1986) Economic aspects of risk assessment in chemical safety. Sci Total Environ 51: 81–124
Kenaga EE (1986) Assessing chemical hazards. Environ Sci Technol 20: 660–662
Mueke W (1987) Risikoabschätzung für Dioxine in der Umwelt. Chemosphere 16: 43–48
Pilz V (1980) Risikoermittlung und Sicherheitsanalysen in der chemischen Technik. Chem Ing Tech 52: 703–711
Pocchiari A et al. (1986) The chemical risk management process in Italy – a case study – the Seveso accident. Sci Total Environ 51: 227–235
Rice AP (1986) Risk management in chemical safety. Sci Total Environ 51: 1–17
Tarkowski S (1986) Data base for risk assessment. Sci Total Environ 51: 19–25
Todhunter JA (1986) Societal considerations in implementing risk management decisions. Sci Total Environ 51: 63–68
World Health Organization (1986) Risk management in chemical safety-conclusions and recommendations. Consultation between experts. Sci Total Environ 51: 261–263
Wilson R (1985) Direct testimony of Richard Wilson. Hearings for the U.S. Congress
Young FE (1987) Risk assessment. Subcommittee on agriculture, U.S. House of Representatives 19 March: 18–21

Medical Risks

Blum AL et al. (1987) The Lugano statements on controlled clinical trials. J Int Med Res 15: 2–22
Charny MC, Farrow SC (1986) Risk targetting: approach to cost-containment. Health Policy 6: 1–10
Evers-Kiebooms G, Cassiman J-J, Van den Berghe H, D'Ydewalle G (eds) (1987) Genetic risk, risk perception, and decisionmaking. Liss, New York
Herman JM (1984) Patients' willingness to take risks in the management of pharyngitis. J Family Practice 19: 767–772
Holzer JF (1984) Current concepts in risk management. Int Anesthesiol Clin 2: 92–116
Mold JW, Stein HF (1986) The cascade effect in the clinical care of patients. N Engl J Med 20 Feb: 512–514
O'Brien B (1986) What are my chances, doctor? a review of clinical risks. Office of Health Education, London
Pauker SG (1987) Decision analysis. N Engl J Med 316: 250–272
Pauker SG, Kassirer JP (1975) Therapeutic decision making: a cost-benefit analysis. N Engl J Med 293: 229–234
Pochin EE (1981) Quantification of risk in medical procedures. Proc R Soc Lond 376a: 87–101
Thompson MS (1986) Willingness to pay and accept risks to cure chronic disease. Am J Public Health 76: 392–396
Weinstein MC, Fineberg HV (1980) Clinical decision analysis. Saunders, Philadelphia

Carcinogens

Ames BN (1983) Dietary carcinogens and anticarcinogens. Science 221: 1256–1264
Ames BN (1984) Unser krebserregendes täglich Brot. Neue Zürcher Zeitung, Beilage Nr. 20: Forschung und Technik, Jan 25
Ames BN et al. (1987) Ranking possible carcinogenic hazards. Science 236: 271–279
Fiering M, Wilson R (1983) Attempts to establish a risk by analogy. Risk Anal 3: 207–216

Gaffey WR (1985) Use of epidemiology in risk assessment. In: Li AP (ed) New approaches in toxicity testing and their application in human risk assessment. Raven, New York, pp 247–251
Hattis DB (1986) The promise of molecular epidemiology for quantitative risk assessment. Risk Anal 6: 181–193
Milvy P (1986) A general guideline for management of risk from carcinogens. Risk Anal 6: 69–79
Montesano R, Tomatis L (1977) Legislation concerning chemical carcinogens in several industrialized countries. Cancer Res 37: 310–316
Ryzin JV (1980) Quantitative risk assessment. J Occup Med 22: 321–326
Smith MV (1984) Use of risk assessment in regulatory decision-making. Food Technol Oct: 114–118

Adverse Drug Reactions

Anonymous (1984) Measuring drug risk: Ciba Geigy's monitoring. Scrip 951: 14–15
Carson FL, Strom BL (1986) Techniques of postmarketing surveillance. Med Toxicol 1: 237–246
Council for International Organizations of Medical Sciences (1986) Monitoring and assessment of adverse drug effects (working group report). CIOMS, Geneva
Faich GA (1986) Adverse-drug-reaction monitoring. N Engl J Med 314: 1589–92
Gingell JC (1986) Non-steroidal anti-inflammatory drugs and serious gastrointestinal adverse reactions – 2. Br Med J 292: 1190–91
Inman WHW (1984) Risks in medical intervention – balancing therapeutic risks and benefits. Pem News 2: 15–36
Inman WHW (1985) Let's get our act together. In: Dukes G (ed) Side effects of drugs annual 9. Elsevier, Amsterdam, pp XV–XX
Karch FE, Lasagna L (1977) Toward the operational identification of adverse drug reactions. Clin Pharmacol Ther 21: 247–254
Keown CF (1985) Contextual effects on people's ratings of seriousness for side effects of prescription drugs. Percept Motor Skills 61: 435–441
Keown CF et al. (1984) Attitudes of physicians, pharmacists and laypersons toward seriousness and need for disclosure of prescription drug side effects. Health Psychol 3: 1–11
Mattison N (1984) Regulatory scene. Pharmaceut Med 1: 13–16
McMahon FG (1983) How safe should drugs be? JAMA 249: 481–482
Napke E (1986) Adverse reactions: some pitfalls and postulates. Center for Study of Drug Development, Boston
Shapiro S (1986) Risks of agranulocytosis and aplastic anemia – their relation to drug use with special reference to analgesics. JAMA 256: 1749–1757
Snell E (1987) How adverse are reactions to medicines? Scrip 1190: 22–23
Tallarida RJ et al. (1984) Non-physicians and physicians assess severity of disease states and adverse drug reactions: application to drug benefit-risk measurement. Pharmaceut Med 1: 41–46
Turner P (1984) Food and drugs: why different approaches to their safety? Lancet 19 May: 1116
Vale JA, Meredith TJ (1986) Acute poisoning due to nonsteroidal anti-inflammatory drugs. Med Toxicol 1: 12–31
Venning GR (1983) Identification of adverse reactions to new drugs I–IV. Br Med J 286: 199–202, 289–292, 365–368, 458–460, 544–547
Venulet J (1984) Functioning of the side effect surveillance system at Ciba-Geigy Basel. Industrie Santé Jan: 49
Venulet J (1987) Informativity of adverse drug reactions data in medical publications. Center for Study of Drug Development (rs 8709), Tufts University, Boston (reprinted from Drug Inform J, 1985, 19: 357–365)

Drug Risks

Anonymous (1984) Measuring drug risk: Ciba-Geigy's monitoring. Scrip 951: 14–15
Anonymous (1987) ABPI issues post marketing surveillance guidelines. Market Lett 7 Nov: 13

Anonymous (1987) Intrauterine devices maker gambles on the informed consumer. Washington Post 13 March
Anonymous (1987) RAD-AR program analyzes risk for Ciba-Geigy. Market Lett 21 Sept: 25
Anonymous (1987) Risk management meeting: conference report, Brighton. Br Med J 294: 1678–79
Azarnoff DL, Herting RL (1984) Drug development: risks and problems. Ann NY Acad Sci 432: 279–285
Borda IT, Bernecker GC (1985) The pharmaceutical industry – drug monitoring by Ciba-Geigy. In: Inman WHW (ed) Monitoring for drug safety. MTP Press Boston, pp 173–200
BPI (ed) (1985) Drugs – potential and risks. BPI, Frankfurt/Main
Brown P (1987) Ciba-Geigy's risk assessment. Scrip 1227: 15
Carroll NV et al. (1986) Perceived risks and pharmacists' generic substitution behavior. J Consumer Aff 20: 36–47
Chetley A, Gilbert A (1986) Problem drugs – introduction. HAI, The Hague, pp 1–4
Council for International Organizations of Medical Sciences (1986) Monitoring and assessment of adverse drug effects (working group report). CIOMS, Geneva
Destevens G (1987) The risks and benefits of drug therapy. Med Res Rev 7: 173–181
Diamond LD, Laurence DR (1985) Product liability in respect of drugs. Br Med J 290: 365–368
Faich GA (1986) Analgetic risks and pharmacoepidemiology. JAMA 256 13: 1788
Haire D (1984) How the FDA determines the "safety" of drugs. National Women's Health Network, Washington D.C.
Hallett C, Dean BC (1984) Bromazepam: acute benefit-risk assessment in general practice. Curr Med Res Opinion 8: 683–688
Heilmann K (1986) Impact of professional and lay media on patients and physicians. Am J Med 80 [Suppl 6a]: 5–7
Inman WHW (1984) Risks in medical intervention – balancing therapeutic risks and benefits. Pem News 2: 15–36
Inman WHW (1985) Let's get our act together. In: Dukes G (ed) Side effects of drugs annual 9. Elsevier, Amsterdam, pp XV–XX
Inman WHW (1987) Requirements for risk-benefit assessment of drugs before withdrawal. Pem News [Suppl] March: 4
Inman WHW (1987) Prescription-event monitoring. Its strategic role in post marketing surveillance for drug safety. Pem News 4: 16–29
Keown CF (1985) Contextual effects on people's ratings of seriousness for side effects of prescription drugs. Percept Motor Skills 61: 435–441
Keown CF, Slovic P, Lichtenstein S (1984) Influence of information about side effects on perceived risk of prescription drugs. In: Winston WJ (ed) Marketing for mental health services. Haworth Press, pp 111–123
Keown CF et al. (1984) Attitudes of physicians, pharmacists and laypersons toward seriousness and need for disclosure of prescription drug side effects. Health Psychol 3: 1–11
Lane DA, Hutchinson TA (1987) The notion of acceptable risk: the role of utility in drug management. J Chronic Dis 40: 621–625
Lasagna L (1987) Postmarketing surveillance of multisource drugs – report of a conference, 9–10 July 1986. Center for the Study of Drug Development, Tufts University ps 8711: 1–58
Laurence DR, Black JW (1978) The medicine you take. Croom Helm, London
McMahon FG (1983) How safe should drugs be? JAMA 249: 481–482
Pedroni G (1982) Drugs and adverse reactions. Pharma Information, Basle
Richard BW (1987) Drug regulation in the United States and the United Kingdom: the depo-prover story. Ann Intern Med 106: 886–891
Shapiro S (1986) Risks of agranulocytosis and aplastic anemia – their relation to drug use with special reference to analgesics. JAMA 256: 1749–1757
Snell E (1987) How adverse are reactions to medicines? Scrip 1190: 22–23
Spitzer WO, Hutchinson T, Lane D (1987) Postmarketing management of drug use: toward rational public policy. Can Med Assoc J 136: 1022–1024
Spivey RN, Lasagna L, Trimble AG (1987) New indication for already-approved drugs: time trends for the new drug application review phase. Clin Pharmacol Ther 41: 368–370
Turner P (1984) Food and drugs: why different approaches to their safety? Lancet 19 May: 1116

Ueberla K (1984) Sicherheit und Risiko im Arzneimittelbereich – Fiktion und Realität. In: Lange S (ed) Ermittlung und Bewertung industrieller Risiken. Springer, Berlin Heidelberg New York
Urquhart J, Heilmann K (1985) Drugs: risk vs benefit. Edition Agrippa, Cologne
Vance MA, Millington WR (1986) Principles of irrational drug therapy. Int J Health Serv 16: 355–362
Venning GR (1984) Priorities in the benefit-risk assessment of new drug. Adverse Drug React Acute Poisoning Rev 3: 113–21
Volans GN (1987) Monitoring the safety of over the counter drugs. Br Med J 295: 797–798
von Wartburg WP (1985) Ten aspects of risk as applied to pharmaceuticals. Ciba-Geigy J 2
Walker SR, Gelzer J et al. (1986) A comparative retrospective analysis of data for short- and long-term animal toxicity studies on 40 pharmaceutical compounds. Center for Study of Drug Development, Boston

29. Subject Index

30. A Handbook of International Data Sources for Drug Benefit/Risk Assessment

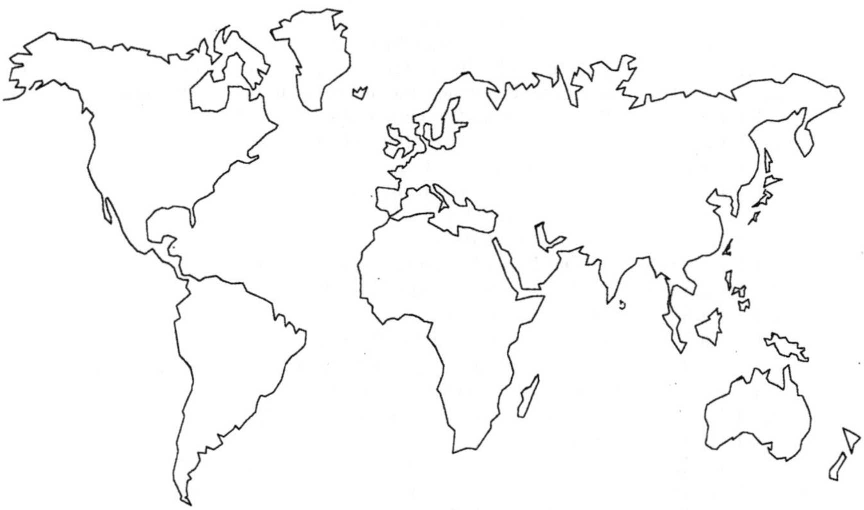

Available through:
Ciba-Geigy Ltd.
Dept. Pharma Politics and Economics
CH-4002 Basle
Switzerland

Table of Contents

Note: United Kingdom data sources will be compiled in a second volume, published at a later date

MIX
Papier aus verantwortungsvollen Quellen
Paper from responsible sources
FSC® C105338
FSC
www.fsc.org

If you have any concerns about our products,
you can contact us on
ProductSafety@springernature.com

In case Publisher is established outside the EU,
the EU authorized representative is:
Springer Nature Customer Service Center GmbH
Europaplatz 3, 69115 Heidelberg, Germany

Printed by Libri Plureos GmbH
in Hamburg, Germany